21 Jan 98

[illegible] best wishes

Walker-Noddey

Migraine — Control and Cure

by

ALEXANDER WALKER-NADDELL
K.St.J., ERD, QHS, FRCS, FRFPS, FSA Scot., FRSA, JP, DL
Consultant Orthopaedic and Neuro Surgeon

Edited by —
ANNIE E. LIVESEY MA

Illustrated by —
ERIC MASTERTON

Published by —
J. R. REID PRINTERS LTD., BLANTYRE, GLASGOW

Typeset in 10 point English Times
on Compugraphic MCS9600 Phototypesetter

ISBN 0 948785 02 0

Typeset, Printed and Published in Scotland by
J. R. Reid Printers Ltd., Blantyre, Glasgow.

Acknowledgements

THIS is the third of my books and all three are closely related in subject matter. They are all concerned with the correction of spinal deformities in order to establish and maintain a good posture, free from pain, throughout the whole length of the spinal column. I cannot stress too strongly the value a good posture contributes to the general appearance, health and wellbeing of all people. This applies in no small measure to migraine sufferers and thus, despite its title, this book is a natural sequel to my first book, 'The Slipped Disc and the Aching Back of Man' * and my second, 'Fight Old Age'. *

Nan Livesey has worked as editor on all three books and I should like to express my gratitude to her. Her hard work, patience and encouragement have enabled me to get the manuscript ready for publication in record time.

I must also thank my printer and publisher, John R. Reid. His professionalism has enabled the last stage of production to proceed smoothly and expeditiously and the accuracy of his team has saved both time and frustration.

* 'The Slipped Disc and the Aching Back of Man' published by J. R. Reid Printers Ltd. in 1985.

* 'Fight Old Age' published by J. R. Reid Printers Ltd. in 1987.

To my late wife, Iris
and my parents
who made it all possible

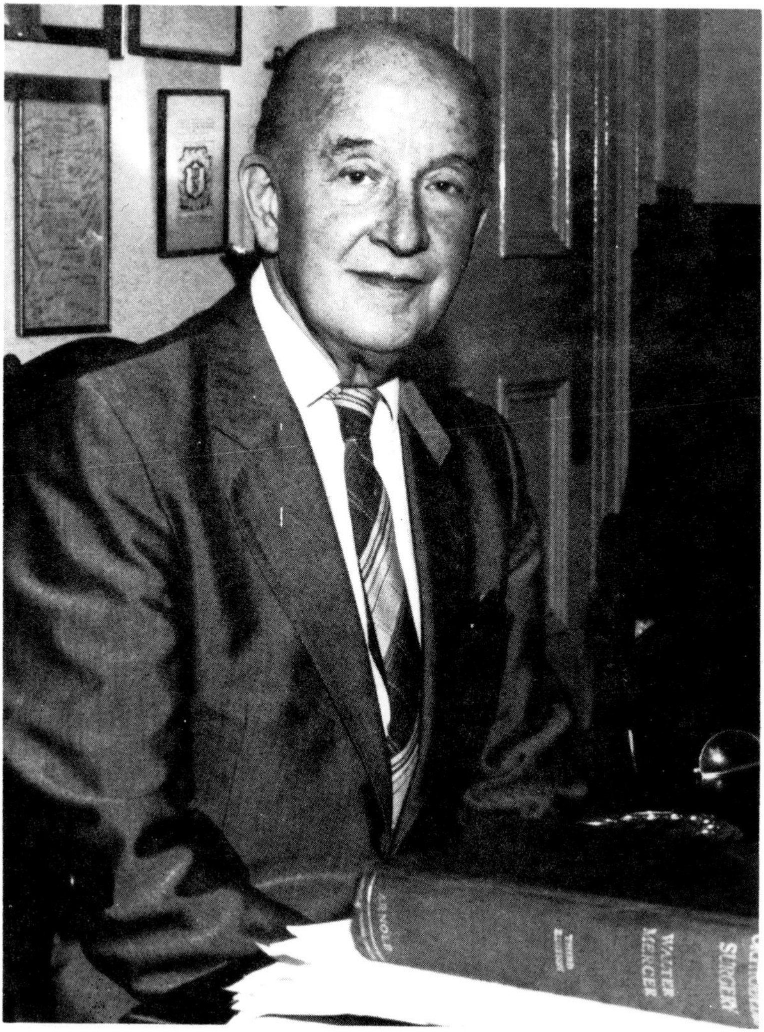

Foreword

By JACK WEBSTER
of The Glasgow Herald

I FIRST encountered Walker Naddell in the 1960s when, as a features writer on the Daily Express, I was pursuing a story about how we would cope with the casualty problem in the unthinkable event of a nuclear war.

The man I should speak to, I was told, was a quiet-spoken neurosurgeon who practised privately in the west end of Glasgow. Alexander Walker Naddell was his name.

But wasn't he the man who specialised in another major topic of the 1960s, the slipped disc? Yes, but he was also the honorary colonel charged with mobilising the massive medical and surgical response to a nuclear war.

A more gentle and unwarlike figure I had seldom met. In the course of our conversations in Glasgow, he discovered that I had been suffering attacks of migraine since I was 18. Now that was interesting.

In his relentless pursuit of remedies for the ills of mankind, he had discovered there was some connection between his treatment for matters like cervical spondylosis and a possible cure for migraine. Patients had come back to tell him that, when he treated them for the one, he seemed to have cured the other.

So he was working backwards to see what it was he was doing which might explain this curious situation. It was still at the experimental stage but would I mind jumping in a taxi the next time I felt an attack coming on? Soon it happened just as it had done several times a year for nearly 20 years of my life.

I was in his room within 15 minutes, still suffering the preliminary loss of sight which always preceded the excruciating headache.

Mr. Naddell set to work on my neck — I had always felt the seat of the problem was somewhere in that region and, as the blindness receded, the customary headache did not materialise. Miraculous! I couldn't believe it. Normally I would have been in bed for the rest of that day at least. What had he done? Well . . . he was working on it.

To cut the story short, I did not have another attack for two or three years. When I was next troubled by migraine, it was less frequent and of a much milder nature. In other words, I could cope with the rest of my day.

I had not been in touch with Mr. Naddell again until I heard he was writing this book. Much had happened, it seemed, and he now felt confident enough to say he had found the cause of migraine and could arrest the symptoms immediately. Medical men are generally cautious about saying they have found a cure — and rightly so. Yet that, in effect, was what Walker Naddell was saying.

I broke the good news in an article in the Glasgow Herald in April, 1989, and Mr. Naddell's claims have been the talk of migraine sufferers ever since.

In the earlier part of this book in particular, he explains his theories in a manner which can be easily understood by the layman. Somehow, it all seems to make sense. Part of the book is more for the consumption of medical people and the author has expressed himself perfectly happy to pass on his expertise to doctors who wish to avail themselves of it.

For the suffering patient, it is a boost to know that relief can be at hand, without the rigmarole of lying in a darkened room for hours on end, having swallowed pills which may or may not have any effect at all.

Mr. Naddell is confident he has found the answer to migraine and has 500 case histories to support his claim. I can only add my own very positive experience — and hope that those days of misery for countless thousands all over the world are within sight of being banished for ever.

CONTENTS

Introduction

THE practice and study of Medicine is always exciting. It is not an exact science so there are always improved methods of treatment to be developed and completely new cures to be discovered. Its practice should never remain static: its practitioners never become complacent. Most new treatments evolve after years of painstaking research but just occasionally one seems to stumble across the solution of an age-old problem quite unexpectedly.

A successful cure for migraine has puzzled doctors for many, many years. When I was a junior surgeon in Glasgow Royal Infirmary the theory was postulated that migraine was caused by the presence of a space-occupying lesion or brain tumour. In order to refute or substantiate this theory I was asked to be present at a number of post mortems of people, known to be chronic migraine sufferers, but who had died from other causes. I attended at least 50 such post mortems but discovered nothing to suggest a brain tumour or the like was present. The theory was discarded and the treatment of migraine not being a surgical problem, was referred back into the hands of the physicians or neurologists. At that time the study of migraine no longer seemed of any great importance to me, as a surgeon.

Some years later my professional career changed and I set up as a private consultant in the West End of Glasgow treating primarily spinal and orthopaedic disorders, specialising in the treatment of the slipped disc condition. Frequently patients suffering from spondylosis and spondylitis of the neck, or cervical vertebral arthritis visited me and I treated them by gentle 'surgical manipulation'. I remember quite clearly one day a patient suffering from cervical spondylosis saying that since my treatment for his neck condition, he had not suffered a single migraine attack although he had previously been a chronic migraine sufferer. I was genuinely pleased for him, but too engrossed in my daily schedule to consider the matter further. However, after many more similar remarks were made from such patients, it dawned on me that this could be no coincidence. Somehow, I was able to cure or at least control migraine but I did not at this stage know **how** my treatment worked or **why** it worked.

Then the real research began. First I read all the standard reference books on migraine. The clinical picture is well known, but not fully understood and thus the methods of treatment to date have been multiple and varied. No method has proved completely effective because only the symptoms are being treated and not the cause of the condition. Until the real cause of an illness has been established the solution can never be completely satisfactory. The treatment of migraine has therefore been empirical and symptomatic. Secondly, I analysed in detail my treatment of spondylitis in the neck and cervical arthritis and especially the position of my hands and fingers during the 'surgical manipulation' that I practise. Thirdly, I studied the anatomy of the head and cervical areas in detail, primarily from that text book of anatomy of all time: Gray's Anatomy and I also returned to the Pathology Department of Glasgow Royal Infirmary in which I had done so much research for the slipped disc condition. During many hours of dissection, I followed the lines of the arteries, veins and nerves in the head and cervical region. Fourthly, I noted in every detail my examination and treatment of 500 cases of chronic migraine sufferers. The clues were all there to solve the problem: the solution was a new treatment of migraine that I describe and explain in the following chapters.

The solution was found by a completely different, radical approach to the subject of migraine, totally disregarding all the current theories that abound today, but relying instead on fundamental research.

The basic premise from which I developed my thesis was that my treatment for cervical disorders also cured migraine. The cervical conditions in question all result in faulty, often fixed forward flexion of the head and neck. My treatment of these involves gentle 'surgical manipulation' during which I gently pull the head backwards and rotate it gently backwards following the arc of a semi-circle or the round part of a capital D.

The second significant factor was that a clinical examination of each migraine sufferer during an attack revealed pronounced dilatation of the common carotid artery on the same side as that affected by the migraine headache. The common carotid artery is the main artery that, dividing into the internal and external carotid arteries, supplies blood respectively to the brain and to the scalp, face and neck. I felt that the behaviour of this large artery held the key to the whole problem of migraine. The big question was what caused this artery to dilate in the first place and how did my treatment for cervical faulty posture reduce the dilatation and control the migraine attack — even it seemed to prevent the occurrence of further attacks.

Thus when I was studying the anatomy of the cervical region both from the text book and by practical dissection, I made particular note of the relationship of the structures in front of the neck when the head was pulled fully forward in the position of faulty posture of the head and also when the head was pulled right back as during my gentle manipulation.

In prolonged forward flexion of the head pressure is exerted by the omo-hyoid muscle in the neck, first on the internal jugular vein and then on to the large common carotid artery that lies just beneath it. The tendonous portion of the muscle acts like a cord cutting right across these vessels. Pressure on the jugular vein gives rise to some cerebral congestion whilst the pressure on the artery causes it to become at first slightly distorted and then constricted, thus obstructing the blood flow to the brain. As we know the brain will not tolerate any interference to its blood supply. A signal from the brain is passed to the heart to pump more quickly and strongly. When this happens the blood surges quickly passed the obstruction on the affected side, dilating all the arteries to the brain via the internal carotid artery and to the face, the side of the head and scalp by the external carotid artery. This sudden dilatation leads to quick flooding of blood to the brain, the side of the face, scalp and neck, as a result of which the patient feels that his head is going to burst and contributes to the particular throbbing headache, typical of migraine.

In the neck the common carotid artery is enclosed in a strong unyielding sheath of cervical fascia. Accompanying the artery are the pneumogastric nerve and the internal jugular vein. When a common carotid artery dilates on one side or the other the accompanying structures i.e. the nerve and vein are compressed against the unyielding fascia. Compression of a nerve gives rise to pain in the area served by that nerve and compression of the vein gives rise to cerebral congestion causing aura, dizziness and possible nausea. From these conditions all the symptoms of the migraine syndrome arise.

Once I had succeeded in isolating the exact cause of migraine, I could confidently perfect a successful treatment.

My treatment falls into two distinct categories. The first is gentle 'surgical manipulation', followed by a training programme of exercises that follow a similar pattern to the manipulation. These are designed, firstly to correct the faulty posture of the head and neck that plays such an important role in triggering off a migraine attack. Secondly, they are designed to exert maximum pressure on the already dilated common carotid artery and thus help to contract the artery and by so doing, control and indeed, at times, halt the migraine attack.

The second part of my treatment is, perhaps the more revolutionary and is, as far as I am aware, a completely new feature in the treatment of migraine. I apply gentle but increased pressure on the dilated common carotid artery with the flat of my thumb on the affected side of the neck to decrease the abnormal blood flow to the brain. Then I extend this treatment by arterial pressure to all accessible arteries in the head and neck area. This is explained in careful detail in Chapter IV, page 63 and should be undertaken only by trained medical practitioners.

My treatment has enormous advantages over the current conventional treatments. It relies on no drugs or diets; it is immediate and thus there is no disruption in the patient's life or work. After the initial course of treatment, if my advice is closely followed, the patient himself can, by simple exercising, control further attacks and prevent them occurring.

CHAPTER I

Current Theories and Treatment of Migraine

THE treatment of migraine seems to have advanced little in the past 50 years. At best it alleviates the patient's symptoms but it still offers no hope of controlling or eradicating the condition.

Migraine is one of the most painful, frustrating conditions known to man. A migraine headache is intense, throbbing and almost unbearable. It is nearly always accompanied by nausea, and/or vomiting and dizziness. Visual disturbances, flashing lights and spots in front of the eyes force patients to lie down in a darkened room as they cannot tolerate bright lights on their eyes. Attacks can occur at any time, making work or play impossible. A migraine sufferer feels that his whole life is dominated by this condition.

And what does modern medicine have to offer such a patient — only pills for sedation and advice to rest in a darkened room for at least 48 hours or longer if the condition does not respond. There is no medication available that permits the patient to carry on living normally during the attacks. The pain of the condition coupled with the frustration of not being able to carry out engagements when planned, make this condition almost insupportable.

The frustration the average migraine sufferer experiences is well illustrated in the case histories I have included in Appendix B (see pages 111-125), most of which have been written by the patients themselves. The letter of Una Orlandi, 44 Parnell Street, Limerick, Ireland, gives a vivid description of the symptoms of migraine. That of Marie Corish, 737 Mosspark Drive, Cardonald, Glasgow, tells of the number and variety of unsuccessful tests and treatments she experienced but most of all, her account records a young life unable to achieve its potential because of migraine. She was advised against going to University and because of her fainting fits became virtually unemployable in certain aspects of her banking career. Mr. J. G. Dawes, 55 Legbourne Road, Louth, Lincolnshire, also describes the various diagnoses and treatments he endured but most significantly, he records how in the absence of a positive diagnosis his symptoms were regarded as psychosomatic. He was referred to a psychiatrist and indeed spent some months in a mental hospital.

These stories demonstrate the need for a new positive diagnosis and real cure for the migraine condition. Migraine sufferers will readily identify with the frustration and despair of these patients before their treatment but must surely take hope from the gratitude these same patients express at the end of their treatment.

Migraine often begins about the age of puberty. The first sign is often innocent enough. A young school girl for example, bright and sitting at the back of the class will discover that she can no longer at times see the blackboard clearly. The teacher will naturally move her to the front of the class and if this does not improve the situation, will alert the parents and suggest the girl be taken to a reputable optician. He will, in good faith, prescribe glasses to correct the disturbance of vision present at that time. Later, however, as these visual symptoms recede, the glasses will prove worthless and may even aggravate the underlying condition and cause headaches. The child will rebel against wearing the glasses and tension between child and parents, supported by teachers, now builds up. As the migraine condition accelerates the girl will suffer increasing bouts of more intense headaches, with nausea and fits of dizziness, even fainting. She will be forced to be absent or sent home from school and spend days in bed. Already other symptoms are being 'built-in' to the migraine syndrome: frustration at having to spend days in bed; mental stress, especially in the bright pupil, caused by missing school work and the fear of falling behind her classmates and tension, even rebellion against parents and teachers, who do not seem to understand or sympathise with her condition.

At this stage the parents will normally seek help from their general practitioner who will see, not only a girl suffering from severe physical symptoms but also, in some considerable state of mental turmoil.

The average family doctor sees many such patients and though many come to him first with this problem as adolescents, migraine may start at any age, and the order in which the symptoms occur varies considerably from case to case. Also, in my experience an equal number of both sexes may be affected and so to redress the balance and for the sake of brevity I will regard my average patient as male.

The doctor, after considering the patient's description of his symptoms, will carry out a normal examination that usually, in these cases, includes a neurological examination testing for the reflexes, and an examination of the eyes with an ophthalmoscope to assess the visual disturbances experienced by the patient. In routine cases he can at this stage suggest that the diagnosis may point to a migraine condition.

However, other conditions show similar clinical signs and the doctor must take these into account before the final diagnosis is made. Every other cause of severe headache must be very carefully considered by the doctor, i.e. a complete differential diagnosis. This is described in detail in Chapter II page 24. The conditions that present the symptoms of an acute headache are numerous and vary in severity from sinusitis to, in extremely rare cases, the presence of a brain tumour.

However, when the differential diagnosis made either by doctor or consultant points to that of migraine then normally pain killing drugs, those developed especially for migraine, are prescribed to be taken in the event of an attack and the patient advised to lie in a darkened room for 24 — 48 hours or until the symptoms subside. Because this treatment is, by no means, ideal medical practitioners have tried to discover what **causes** the attacks to prevent a recurrence. 'Prevention is better than cure', is extremely apt when currently considering the migraine syndrome.

Theories concerning the cause of migraine are various and fragmented suggesting an absence of a positive proven theory. The main theories that seem in vogue today can be described under three headings: diet, stress, hormonal imbalance.

Current Theories of the Cause of Migraine

1. Diet

Some doctors suggest that various food products, like chocolate and cheese, and drinks containing alcohol or caffeine are responsible for the onset of attacks. Thus they prescribe a life-long diet, avoiding or limiting such substances to prevent the onset of an attack.

2. Stress

Many doctors think stress is the prime factor that causes migraine. The general practitioner will usually very patiently ask the migraine sufferer to describe his lifestyle and try to discover if he is under great mental strain at school or work or if there have been any emotional upsets in his family or social life. If he feels it necessary he may prescribe mild tranquilisers and will almost certainly counsel the patient to adopt a less hectic or stressful lifestyle if this seems appropriate. If the doctor or consultant concludes that the symptoms and case history suggest a psychological or psychiatric undertone, then he will advise getting help from a psychiatrist, or even a hypnotist, to try to discover why these attacks persist. The psychiatrist may conclude after many sessions with the patient that the symptoms have a direct bearing on a psychological problem within the patient, arising from some emotional upset in his youth, or alternatively tension within his family. He may suggest they arise from mental stress if the patient seems overworked or over anxious about work. If this is the case he may advise against the patient pursuing higher education at, say, a University or in the case of an adult against accepting promotion at work, fearing the patient would be incapable of assuming further responsibilities. Considering that many migraine patients have a high IQ this seems to be a considerable waste of potentiality, often resulting, later on, in a feeling of failure, lack of fulfilment and loss of self assurance. The psychiatrist may even suggest that the attacks are brought on by auto-suggestion when the patient is forced up against an unpleasant task or an examination, for example. This again will undermine self confidence and also cause great resentment within the patient who has worked and studied hard to overcome an obstacle or pass an examination.

In all these circumstances psychiatric therapy will be recommended and very often a course of valium or some such medication will be prescribed. Such medicines are at the extreme end of the spectrum; they interfere with concentration and the quality of mental work undertaken and the associated grave dangers of addiction cannot be overstated.

3. Hormonal Imbalance

Some medical practitioners attribute the cause of migraine to hormonal imbalance, especially when treating female patients.

The general practitioner at the first consultation usually notes whether the attacks are associated in adolescents with the time of menstruation or in the older woman with the menopause and will prescribe hormonal therapy if necessary, accordingly. If a female patient is taking the oral contraceptive pill, then he may suggest a variant or to discontinue taking it for a time.

Some consultants believe that hormonal imbalance is the key factor in the migraine syndrome and so after discovering from the patient's history that the G.P.'s hormonal therapy has proved unsuccessful he may refer the patient to a gynaecologist. This consultant, after a complete examination may find one ovary is enlarged due to an ovarian cyst. He will advise the cyst or possibly the ovary be removed in the hope that the symptoms of dizziness, fainting and nausea will disappear. This is rarely successful. If the cyst is on the right side of the abdomen then the surgeon would investigate the condition of the appendix and if it is at all inflamed he will usually remove this at the same time.

Tests, investigations, even minor operations, may continue over months and years because if the patient is a genuine migraine sufferer the attacks will persist in both frequency and severity. Thus at each stage he is driven back to try to get more help from any medical, or even alternative source, that seems to offer the possibility of a cure.

The patient may also feel some concern at the number of pills he is taking — often up to 10 a day. He may even experience an upset stomach with loss of appetite as a result of the gastric irritation caused by the pills.

All hospital investigations are very relevant if the clinical features the patient presents suggest in any way that the condition is pathological. The negative results give peace of mind to both patient and consultant and should always be undertaken if there is any doubt at all about the cause of the patient's illness.

However fortunately, these serious conditions are relatively rare among typical migraine sufferers and the relief experienced by the negative results soon turns to frustration when the attacks continue as before. The only treatment on offer is medication in the form of pills and rest in a darkened room for 24 — 48 hours during an attack. Neither consultant nor doctor can suggest any alternative treatment. All too often in these circumstances the patient is simply told that he will have to live with this regime for the rest of his life (or at least until late middle age). Patients tell me at this point they feel condemned to a life sentence of suffering and despair.

Meantime, frustration, tension, rebellion in the young, are having a disastrous effect on the personality of the patient and are equally damaging to his quality of life by denying him the opportunities that life in other circumstances would offer. He is afraid to assume responsibilities for fearing of letting people down at the last moment. His self esteem is in grave danger of being ruined.

The sheer diversity of the four theories put forward as the cause of migraine seems to indicate a lack of positivity. No single true cause has been established and in my opinion until this has been attained, no cure will be completely effective.

I frankly do not agree with any of these current theories and my reasons will become virtually self evident when I have established in Chapter III my own proven theory as to the cause of migraine. I explain my reasoning in some detail in the same chapter, see page 42.

Current Treatment of Migraine

Current treatment, in the absence of a positive proven theory treats only the symptoms of the condition and quite often these are still slow to subside. As already indicated it consists of medication prescribed, usually in the form of a pill, to alleviate the severe headache and to help the patient relax, and if possible, sleep. The doctor or consultant also advises patients to rest in a darkened room for 24 — 48 hours during an attack.

This form of treatment is of great value to the patient. A migraine sufferer usually cannot bear any form of bright light on his eyes and so a darkened room helps to clear away the visual disturbances or aura nearly always associated with the condition. Also when a patient is lying down, especially on his back, the arterial pressure to the neck and brain is greatly reduced. The diminished activity will automatically, but slowly, reduce the blood flow to the head and neck. Thus all symptoms will, in time, slowly subside, but only temporarily.

Whilst I agree that this current form of treatment is beneficial, **my own treatment** (described in Chapter IV, page 45) **has overwhelming advantages.** It is simple to administer and the results of my treatment are immediate. No medication in the form of drugs is required, so there can be no possible side effects. No dietary requirements are necessary and the patient no longer has to shut himself away in a darkened room. There are therefore no further disruptions in the patient's occupation or lifestyle. Most importantly when the patient realises the true cause of migraine as I shall describe it, he can henceforth avoid any further attacks throughout his life. Thus my treatment can, not only immediately arrest the symptoms of migraine but also can control and in many cases, completely eradicate the condition.

CHAPTER II

The Description and Diagnosis of the Migraine Syndrome

THE name 'Migraine' is derived from the term 'hemicrania', which means pain or aching on one side of the head. Classically, it is defined as a paroxysmal headache usually unilateral, as the name suggests, but not invariably so. It occurs at irregular intervals usually with visual disturbances, nausea, vomiting, and other disorders of cerebral function. Because of the nausea and vomiting, it was, at times referred to as 'sick headache', 'bilious headache' or 'nervous headache'. Frequently areas of numbness occur in various parts of the neck and face and occasionally in the arms and fingers.

Historically, migraine is a condition which has affected men and women throughout the ages and records reveal that it is a condition that strikes people in all walks of life, both rich and poor alike.

Migraine does not shorten life. It is not, as a rule, a killer disease and this reassurance should be stressed to every patient at the first consultation before one embarks on treatment. The acute severe throbbing headache of migraine is possibly the worst headache of all and to say the least, it is in many cases soul destroying, hanging like a dark cloud over the afflicted individuals. The suddenness and irregularity of severe attacks cause work schedules and social engagements to be upset. If the condition is not checked a state of chronic nervous exhaustion may result which severely impedes concentration. Thus migraine often disrupts the patient's working life and indeed may erode and destroy family and social life also. It comes high in the list of causing man hours lost per year, affecting approximately 10% to 15% of the population and, as sufferers usually have a high I.Q., the frequent loss of their skills must have an indirect effect on our country's economy. It would seem therefore, that a successful cure for migraine would be of real benefit to the prosperity of the country as well as more importantly to the well-being of those who suffer from it.

Migraine may begin in childhood, but more commonly it develops during adolescence and does not abate in intensity until past middle age.

The onset of the migraine syndrome differs from case to case and the order in which the symptoms occur varies considerably. Many patients feel faint and dizzy whilst others may experience nausea as the early symptom. This gives rise to extreme pallor with a feeling of chilliness and cold feet. The skin will feel cold and clammy with varying degrees of perspiration. Very commonly bright or black spots in front of the eyes or **aura** will be the warning of an impending attack.

The patient often seems restless and mentally depressed with a fear of impending evil. He may feel a tingling sensation in his fingers and toes. There may be a twitching of facial muscles with a possible disturbance of speech which may last for many minutes. These symptoms are succeeded by a severe headache which generally commences in one spot and gradually involves one half or the whole of the head. The attack is usually terminated by a feeling of nausea and possible vomiting after which the headache slowly passes away.

It must be stressed however, that every patient suffers different symptoms, occurring in a different order. Variation in the extent, severity and duration of the symptoms is great and considerable overlapping of symptoms also occurs. Sometimes a patient will experience only **some** of the symptoms and even the most common symptom — the throbbing headache, may not be present. Such patients may experience aura, disturbance of sight, even some patchy numbness but yet have no pain in the head. Any form of work is still impossible and nausea and vomiting may or may not accompany the aura. The term 'syndrome' therefore is aptly applicable to the condition of migraine for it embraces the whole group of signs and symptoms that collectively indicate or characterise the affliction.

The migraine syndrome may be divided into four main categories:

1. Headache (Hemicrania)
2. Aura
3. Nausea and vomiting
4. Cerebral disturbance

1. Headache or Hemicrania

The headache is usually unilateral, as the name suggests, and commonly starts at the base of the skull at the back of the neck (the post occipital area). Pain also occurs above the eye-brows (the supra orbital area) and extends upwards to form a tight band over the top of one side or other of the head. At times the headache is so agonising together with a feeling that the head is going to burst, that it is not unknown for a patient in this state to keep striking his head against a wall in the hope of getting relief. The headache waxes in intensity and becomes severe, being aggravated by movement, strong light and noise. It eases and becomes less intense in the recumbent position. It is boring and throbbing in character and may become bilateral when at its maximum. Patients will also complain of pain and throbbing in the temporal region. They may also experience twitching of muscles in the face, usually in the region of the upper jaw. Pain may also be present at the base of the neck and may extend over the shoulder into the arm, with a pins and needles sensation in the fingers and possible cramping of the hand and fingers.

2. **Aura**

Aura is a sensation, such as of a cold breeze or flashes of light that precedes the onset of nervous disorders. The patient may be suddenly conscious of a bright illuminated and shimmering spot on one side of the field of vision. This tends to enlarge and to open out into a curved zig-zag figure, the so-called 'fortification spectrum'. The figure flickers before him and may be accompanied by the prese- of black dots in the field of vision. At times a dimming or partial blotting out of the field of vision occurs which sometimes amounts to a hemianopia (blindness for one half of the field of vision in one or both eyes).

Pain may also be present in and around the eye socket.

3. **Nausea**

Nausea may be the first sign of an impending migraine, but usually it comes on immediately after the onset of hemicrania or headache. In some cases nausea often with vomiting may herald the termination of the migraine attack. Though nausea nearly always occurs as part of the migraine syndrome, vomiting may or may not occur and rarely does active vomiting occur without prior nausea.

4. **Cerebral Congestion and Disturbance**

Cerebral congestion gives the patient a feeling of light headedness with nausea and/or active vomiting. The patient may feel so dizzy that he has to hold on to something to prevent falling down. In some cases the patient may faint which, at times, may resemble the onset of an attack of epilepsy. Cerebral congestion will also cause chilliness, shivering and bouts of perspiration often associated with nausea.

DIAGNOSIS OF THE MIGRAINE SYNDROME OR CONDITION

A firm diagnosis of any medical problem is made on the combined assessment of the symptoms a patient presents and the clinical signs manifest during the examination of the patient by the doctor or consultant.

At the first consultation I always take a very careful history of the patient's condition starting off with the symptoms that he has at that particular time. I ask when this particular attack started and what, in his opinion, caused it. I then carefully go into the history of the first ever attack of this problem, recording every symptom in detail.

As I have already indicated in Chapter I, page 17 many conditions present the symptom of an acute headache, possibly accompanied by nausea and/or aura. The doctor must satisfy himself that he has taken every factor into account before he makes a firm diagnosis. In other words, he must make a complete differential diagnosis.

The Differential Diagnosis of a Severe Headache

1. Acute headache will accompany a fever, but the normal checking of temperature, pulse and respiration if found to be normal over a period of a day or so, will eliminate most febrile conditions.

2. If it is a first consultation and the doctor's examination shows some nasal congestion then he may relate the headache to sinusitis, the result of a viral infection, and prescribe an inhalant and/or an antibiotic to clear the congestion and possibly resulting headache.

3. Some patients may complain of stiffness and/or pain at the base of the neck which may radiate upwards into the head and/or

downwards into the shoulder area. There may be a tendency to the development of a 'Dowager's hump' with a prominence of the posterior cervical processes, usually C.5/6/7/D1 or even a flattening of the normal lower cervical lordosis. In such cases the patient may be referred to an orthopaedic surgeon.

4. If not undertaken already the doctor may suggest that the patient has an eye test by an optician to make quite sure the visual disturbances he has described are not indicating eye strain or even serious disorders of the eye.

5. If the patient complains that he actually falls in fainting fits at the beginning of the attacks then the doctor will almost certainly refer him as soon as possible to a consultant for further investigation. Similarly if the attacks do not lessen or even become more frequent then the patient on a succeeding visit will normally be sent to a consultant, either a physician or consultant neurologist, preferably one who specialises in the migraine syndrome.

6. Most importantly, if a particular attack does not subside and the visual disturbances are constant with no relief being obtained from rest in a darkened room, then the doctor would certainly refer the patient to a consultant without delay. He would, in these circumstances, suspect the possible presence of a space-occupying lesion within the skull, for in this case the visual disturbances become permanent and progressive.

The consultant will examine the patient, including checking his chest and lungs, his central nervous system and his vascular system including heart and vessels. In routine cases he will confirm that the patient is suffering from the migraine syndrome.

7. However, if there is any doubt about the nature and extent of the headache and visual disturbances he will propose further tests to make absolutely sure no brain tumour or space-occupying lesion is present. A straight x-ray of the skull will indicate if further investigation is required, whereupon he will advise a brain scan to be undertaken. At the same time an x-ray of the chest should be done to make sure the lungs are clear.

8. If the patient regularly has fainting fits, especially those that last 5 — 10 minutes, then he would recommend the patient have an

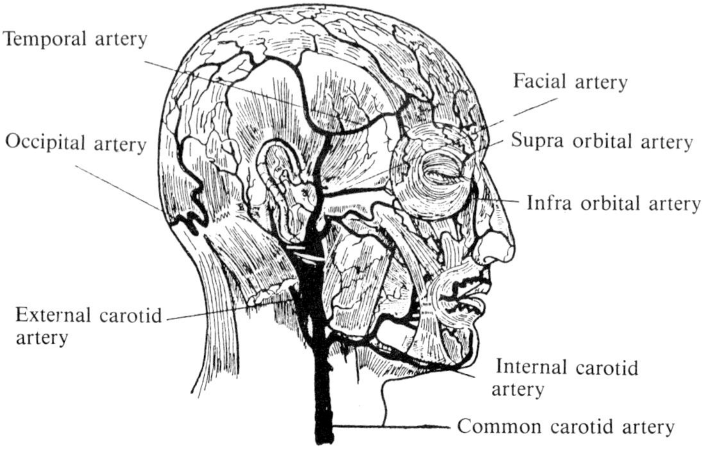

Diagram showing the superficial arteries of the neck, face and head.

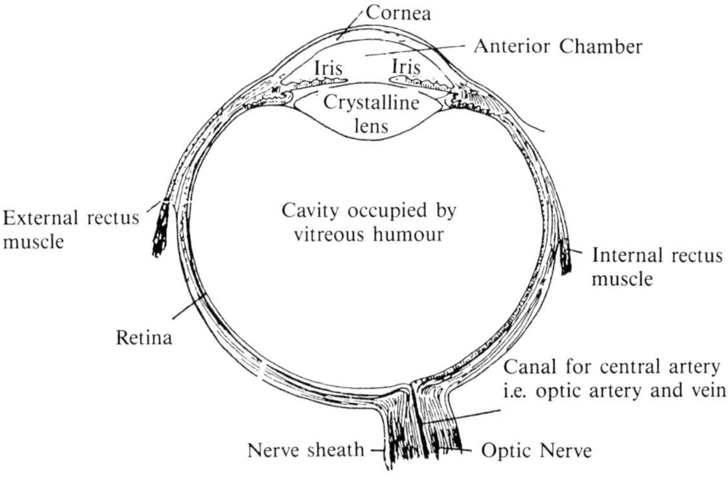

A horizontal section of the eyeball.

electro-encephalogram in case the systems indicate the onset of epilepsy or other brain malfunction.

9. An ECG may also be advised to check the condition of the heart.

10. A sample of blood is often taken and sent to the pathology department to exclude the possibility of glandular fever or any other infection.

However, in routine cases or when the tests prove negative the doctor or consultant would consider that the throbbing headache, the aura and cerebral disturbances the patient presents would point to a diagnosis of a migraine syndrome. This diagnosis would then be confirmed by a clinical examination that should reveal the following signs.

The Clinical Signs of the Migraine Syndrome

1. **Dilatation of the common carotid artery** on the side of the neck. I usually examine the patient either sitting or standing with his back towards me. The artery is easily palpated between the lower borders of the mandible and the upper quarter of the anterior aspect of the sterno-mastoid muscle. On the affected side the common carotid artery will be found to be dilated and pulsing very strongly in time with the normal regular heart beat. The use of the stethoscope over the common carotid artery on the affected side will reveal a much stronger pulse beat than on the unaffected side. I have now adopted this as a routine standard method of examining patients.

2. **Dilatation of the temporal artery** which is easily seen pulsating in time with the heartbeat in the superficial temporal region. This may occur on one side or more rarely on both. The temporal vein may stand out prominently (see Appendix A, page 105).

3. **Tender Eye Ball** The patient is asked to close his eyes. Slight pressure on the eyeballs when migraine is present will cause slight pain and the eyeball itself will feel firm and hard.

4. **The ophthalmoscopic examination** of the fundus or back of the eye in migraine sufferers may reveal some dilatation of the arteries on the affected side. Slight haemorrhages of the fundus may be present as a result of this dilatation. When the migraine condition subsides the artery dilatation in the fundus of the eye will contract to normal.

5. **Faulty Cervical Posture** Most, if not all, migraine sufferers hold their head in a varying degree of forward flexion. This faulty posture of the head and neck is actually, in my opinion the root cause of migraine and will be explained in detail in the following chapter (see Chapter III, page 33). During the examination the headache may be intensified by increasing the forward flexion of the head. By this movement the already dilated artery is yet further dilated, thus increasing the throbbing headache.

In the older age groups the faulty posture often develops into a fixed forward flexion of the head with a loss of mobility in the cervical or neck area and accompanying pain at the base of the neck which may radiate upwards into the head and downwards into the shoulder area. Pain is usually experienced with any backward extension of the head and there is considerable loss of rotation of the head. Audible creaking noises are heard when these movements are attempted.

During the examination the patient is asked to remove clothing from the neck, shoulders and arms. I then carefully examine the cervical and upper dorsal regions for any spinal deformity: for example, deviation of the cervical spinal column to one side or the other i.e. scoliosis or more precisely in the neck, torticollis. There may be undue prominence of the posterior cervical processes, usually C.5/6/7/D1 giving rise to a slight to moderate 'Dowager's hump'. There may be flattening of the normal lower cervical hollow or lordosis curve giving rise to some forward fixed flexion of the head with rounding of the shoulders. Cervical spondylosis or spondylitis, which involves contraction of the intrinsic muscles and ligaments of the cervical area, is quite common in the over forties. As a rule this can be confirmed by a radiologist who may report slight to moderate degenerative arthritic change. Many such patients are advised by their doctor or consultant to wear a surgical collar and take antiarthritic drugs to relieve the pain and clear up the arthritis. I believe the use of a surgical collar to be misguided. It is uncomfortable to wear and often gives the patient a sense of claustrophobia. More importantly its use often causes muscle disuse atrophy and further loss of movement in the neck.

If the pain is intense and has shown no sign of abating with such treatment and especially if torticollis is present, I would immediately suspect the presence of a cervical disc lesion which is pressing on a nerve root. Arthritis of the anterior aspects of the vertebra bodies never gives rise to nerve root pain. I have attended over 100 post mortems and in not a single case was there evidence of arthritic change with osteophytes growing in the neural canals.

The commonest sites of cervical disc lesions which would give rise to torticollis and migraine are between the vertebral bodies of C.3/4, 4/5 and 5/6.

My diagnosis and treatment of a cervical disc lesion has been described in great detail in my book, 'The Slipped Disc and the Aching Back of Man'. * The treatment for the detachment of the disc would be undertaken immediately. As the torticollis is a direct, secondary result of a cervical disc lesion correct posture will not be attained until the disc has been detached. It follows that if, as I maintain migraine is directly related to faulty posture of the head, then correct alignment of the cervical spinal column is essential to the control and cure of the migraine condition.

* 'The Slipped Disc and the Aching Back of Man' published by J. R. Reid Printers Ltd. in 1985.

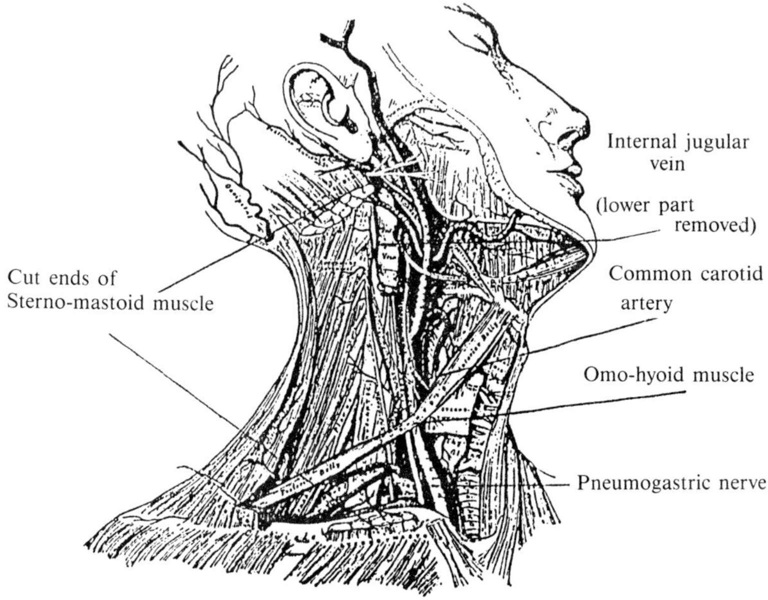

Diagram to show the relationship of the sterno-mastoid and the omo-hyoid muscles to the common carotid artery, jugular vein and pneumogastric nerve.

CHAPTER III

My Analysis of the Cause of Migraine and my Evaluation of the Current Theories

IT CAN be seen from the clinical signs and symptoms of migraine just described in the previous chapter that all migraine sufferers are affected by arterial dilatation. I have not the slightest doubt that migraine is the direct result of dilatation of the arteries in the neck and head. It starts in the neck and extends upwards to the superficial aspects of the head and internally to the brain.

The artery to be first affected is the common carotid artery which is the main artery that supplies the blood from the ventricles of the heart to the head and neck. This artery divides into two main branches, the internal carotid which supplies all the brain and the external carotid that supplies all the face, the neck and the scalp.

Most arteries in the body run in close proximity to a vein and a nerve. Many arteries and their branches run with an accompanying nerve and a vein through bony canals. The supra and infra orbitals passing above and below the eye are examples of such arteries. Others, again with an accompanying nerve and vein are enclosed in a tough unyielding fibrous tube or sheath. This is true of the common carotid artery that is contained in a sheath derived from deep cervical fascia which also encloses the pneumogastric nerve and the internal jugular vein (see diagram opposite). Finally, some superficial arteries, the temporal at the side of the forehead, for example, with accompanying nerves and veins are together covered by a tough, unyielding, fibrous fascia or membrane.

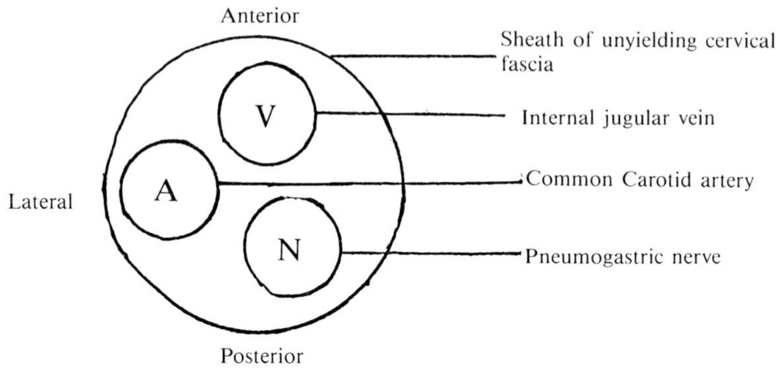

1. Diagram of the normal positioning of the common carotid artery, the internal jugular vein and the pneumogastric nerve.

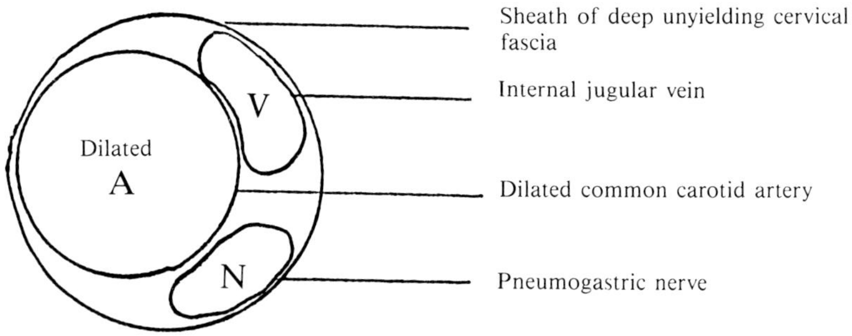

Note the dilatation of the common carotid artery pressing on the internal jugular vein and the pneumogastric nerve.

2. Diagram to show pressure of dilated common carotid artery on pneumogastric nerve and internal jugular vein.

In all these circumstances the three structures, i.e. the artery, vein and nerve are contained in a restricted space, incapable of expansion. Thus, when the artery dilates, it compresses both its accompanying nerve and vein (see diagram opposite).

Pressure on a nerve by a dilated artery will give rise to extreme pain in the area supplied by that nerve. In the case of migraine, this causes the characteristic severe headache, the precise location of pain depending on which nerve is being compressed. For example pressure on the temporal nerve will give rise to pain at the temple. Most importantly, pressure on the pneumogastric nerve, that supplies the oesophogus, or stomach with motor fibres (see Appendix A, pages 97-99) is responsible to a great extent for the symptoms of nausea and/or vomiting nearly always present in a migraine attack.

Pressure on the accompanying vein by a dilated artery will give rise to a disturbance of venous return from the brain, thus causing varying degrees of cerebral congestion. The artery meanwhile continues to pump blood more vigorously in order to overcome the degree of cerebral congestion. Thus the failure of venous return from the brain will be increased even more, producing even more cerebral congestion. This leads to symptoms such as dizziness and aura and may contribute to the symptoms of nausea and vomiting.

Cerebral congestion not only affects the motor area of the cerebral cortex of the brain but also its sensory area. The pressure on the sensory cortex of the brain will give rise to a variety of sensory disturbances affecting any part of the body. For example it may give rise to the chilliness and slight perspiration associated with nausea.

In my opinion in the case of migraine sufferers, **the dilatation of the arteries is caused by faulty posture.** The whole head of these patients is held in slight to moderate forward flexion. This is usually a direct result of the patient's occupation or profession which involves prolonged forward stooping of the head. Thus secretaries, students, writers, draughtsmen or surgeons etc. may be particularly affected. In actual fact, most every day activities involve **some** forward flexion of the head, even eating, resting, sleeping. However, when a person's occupation demands **constant** forward flexion of the head and neck throughout his working life, then he may adopt a fixed forward position of his head and neck with flattening of the normal cervical lordosis or curve.

Continuous faulty posture of the head and neck results in mechanical pressure being exerted by the sterno-mastoid muscles of the neck on to the vessels that lie beneath them. This pressure is

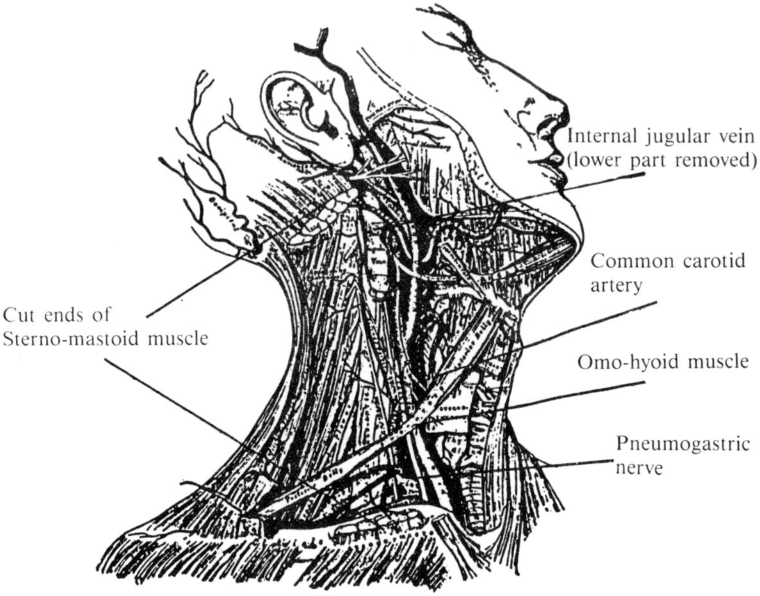

Diagram to show the relationship of the sterno-mastoid and the omo-hyoid muscles to the common carotid artery, jugular vein and pneumogastric nerve.

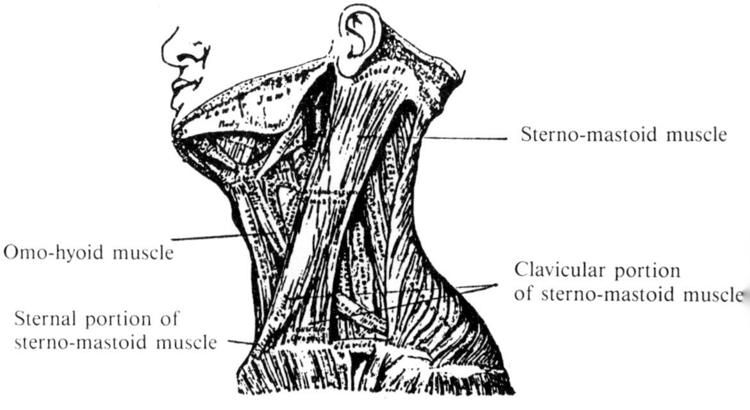

Diagram to show the sterno-mastoid and the omo-hyoid muscles.

aggravated, especially when the head is bent over sideways as well as forwards, by the mechanical pressure of the central tendon of the omo-hyoid muscle that lies beneath the sterno-mastoid muscles and cuts across the sheath containing the jugular vein, the common carotid artery and the pneumogastric nerve, (see diagram opposite and Appendix A, page 79 for the relationship of the omo-hyoid muscle to these structures). This pressure is exerted first on to the jugular vein, causing some cerebral congestion and secondly on to the common carotid artery. The compression of the common carotid artery leads to distortion and constriction of the artery causing a diminution of the blood supply to the brain, known as cerebral ischaemia. The brain will not tolerate any interference to its blood supply and so the heart begins to beat more strongly to pump more blood up to the brain. This results in an immediate dilatation of initially the common carotid artery, and then of all the arteries to the head, to overcome the initial diminution of the blood supply to the brain (i.e. cerebral ischaemia) caused by the stricture. The dilated arteries tightly confined in unyielding fascial membrane, fibrous sheaths or bony canals cause compression of their accompanying nerves and veins that results in pain and cerebral disturbance and all the symptoms of the migraine syndrome.

In my study of 500 patients I noted that the great majority of them had migraine on the left side. I realised that most people are right handed and wondered if this was the cause. When people write or work with their hands they naturally tilt their heads to the opposite side of the working hand. This would cause extra pressure on the common carotid artery on that side, and thus possibly set up dilatation of the arteries.

I think, however, the more likely cause is inherent in the anatomy of the 10th or pneumogastric nerve and that of the internal jugular vein (see Appendix A, page 99). The course of the 10th or pneumogastric nerve is different on the two sides of the body. On the left side it enters the chest between the common carotid and subclavian arteries. Thus a dilated common carotid artery may readily cause pressure on the pneumogastric nerve leading to symptoms of nausea and possible vomiting. On the right side, however, the 10th nerve does not pass in such close proximity to the common carotid artery and thus pressure on the nerve is less likely to occur. Also, (see Appendix A, page 100) as the nerve ascends the neck area, it gives off more numerous oesophageal branches on the left side than on the right side. This may also have some bearing on the fact that migraine is more common on the left side.

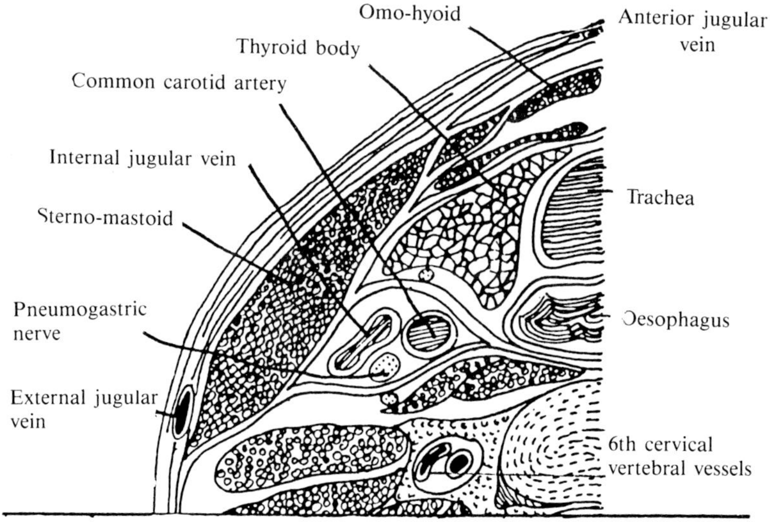

Section of the neck at about the level of the sixth cervical vertebra, showing the arrangement of the deep cervical fascia.

Similarly the course of the internal jugular vein is different on each side of the neck (see Appendix A, page 109). At the base of the neck the vein on the right side is placed a little distance from the common carotid artery but on the left side it usually lies over the artery at its lower part. A dilated common carotid artery can more readily compress the vein on the left side because of its proximity to the vein and thus interfere with the venous return from the brain, head and neck.

A Summary showing how all the Migraine Symptoms arise from ARTERIAL DILATATION

1. Dilatation of the Common Carotid Artery

After the compression and stricture caused by faulty posture, the common carotid artery, to overcome the initial ischaemia, then dilates within its unyielding fibrous sheath. This dilatation causes pressure on both its accompanying pneumogastric nerve and the internal jugular vein. Compression of the pneumogastric or vagus nerve gives rise to the symptoms of nausea and/or vomiting whilst compression of the internal jugular vein interferes with the return flow of venous blood from the brain and neck, causing varying degrees of cerebral congestion. This congestion gives rise to visual disturbances, aura, a feeling of dizziness and instability.

At times, the dilated common carotid artery will press on some segment of the brachial plexus of nerves, giving rise to atypical brachial neuritis. Pain is experienced at the base of the neck on the affected side, often extending into the arm with referred pain in the region of the elbow. The condition may extend to the fingers, resulting in cramping numbness of the hand and possible twitching of the fingers.

Constriction of the common carotid artery, followed by swift compensatory dilatation will result almost immediately in dilatation of **all the other arteries in the neck and head,** including the brain. Those that are of importance in the treatment of migraine are listed below. These are selected because they permit easy access for treatment by mechanical pressure on the dilated artery. Nevertheless, it must be stressed that **all arteries** in the affected side are dilated

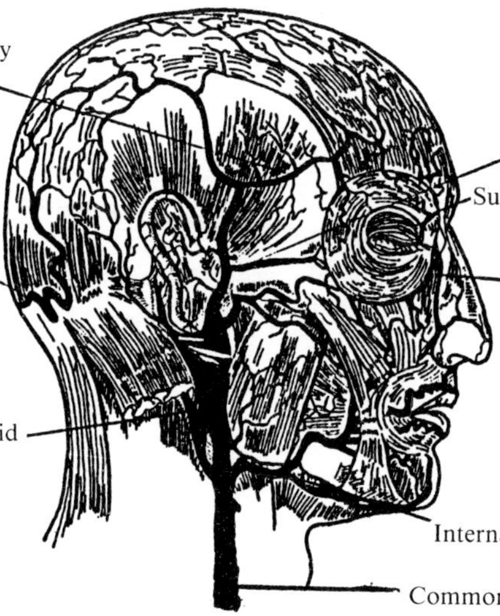

Diagram showing the superficial arteries of the neck, face and head.

and every symptom in the migraine syndrome is directly due to the pressure of a dilated artery on its accompanying nerve and vein. For example, the lingual artery mechanically pressing on the lingual nerve causes a pins and needles sensation of the tongue.

2. **Dilatation of the Posterior Occipital Artery**

This causes pain by pressure on the post occipital nerve, which in turn, causes spasm of the muscular part of the post occipital fascia, the aponeurosis. This tension on the fascia extends upwards to the top of the head (i.e. the vertex).

3. **Dilatation of the Supra Orbital Artery**

This artery emerges at the medial side of the eyebrow. Pain is caused in this area by the pressure of the supra orbital artery on the supra orbital nerve. The nerve pressure causes the supra orbital muscles to go into spasm. This in turn causes the aponeurosis or fascia in this area to become very tight extending upwards to the top of the head. In other words the whole of the occipital fascia or aponeurosis is now pulled like a tight band over the affected side of the head. This accounts for the feeling of the patient that his whole skull is being tightly compressed together with a sensation that his head feels as if it will burst.

4. **Dilatation of the Inferior Orbital Artery**

This causes pressure on the inferior orbital nerve, resulting in pain in the region of the lower eye socket (the infra-orbital area) with occasional twitching of the upper cheek and/or lower eyelid.

5. **Dilatation of the Temporal Artery**

This causes pressure on the temporal nerve, giving rise to acute pain at the temple, with twitching of the skin in the temporal region.

6. **Dilatation of the Facial Artery**

This causes pressure on the facial nerve, leading to pain in an area just in front of the ear and extending in a parallel line just above the upper jaw. With this pain, muscle twitching at the side of the face commonly occurs.

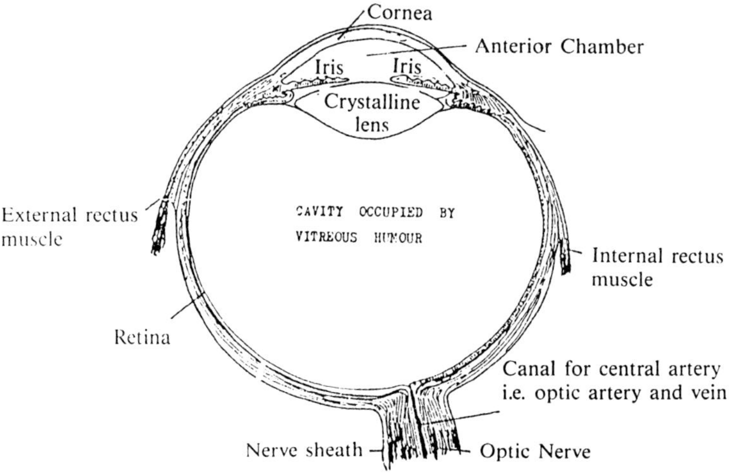

A horizontal section of the eyeball.

7. **Dilatation of the Optic Artery**

This causes pressure on the optic nerve, giving rise to pain behind the eye, with a very acute splitting headache over the eye on the affected side. It may cause very slight haemorrhages in the fundus of the eye, causing blurring of vision, loss of partial field of vision (hemianopia), black spots in front of the eye and many features of aura. Some of these symptoms will also have a definite relationship to the cerebral congestion caused by arterial pressure on the internal jugular vein.

These symptoms collectively form the whole migraine syndrome, but all may not be present at any one time in any individual. Though these features have been tabulated to form a convenient clinical picture there is a considerable amount of variation and overlapping of symptoms. It should never be forgotten that when dilatation occurs it can affect **every** artery of the head, neck and brain. However in migraine it is commonly only one side of the head, face and neck, that is affected and hence the name 'hemicrania', but occasionally both sides of the head and neck may be affected.

(N.B. It should be noted that the description given above relates to one side of the head and neck only. All the structures listed, together with accompanying nerves and veins, are described and illustrated in Appendix A.)

MY EVALUATION OF CURRENT THEORIES

In the light of this exposition of my theory, I should briefly like to give my professional opinion on the more popularly held beliefs about migraine referred to in Chapter I, page 17.

1. Diet

Many migraine sufferers relate the onset of a migraine attack, especially if nausea is experienced, with the food and drink taken prior to the attack. Some medical practitioners support this theory and hence many diets excluding hot tea, coffee, chocolate, cheese, alcohol etc. are prescribed **for life** to avoid further attacks. I believe such abstention to be totally unnecessary because, in my opinion, the onset of nausea and/or vomiting, frequently an early sign of a migraine attack, is a direct result of the mechanical pressure of the dilated common carotid artery on the pneumogastric nerve and on the internal jugular vein. Thus the consumption of these various foods can have no bearing whatsoever on the migraine syndrome. The intake of alcoholic beverages or those containing caffeine may **marginally precipitate an impending attack** but it **cannot cause** it. These products do cause slight dilatation of the arteries. If the artery is already dilated, then the increased dilatation may cause extra pressure on the pneumogastric nerve sufficient to cause nausea and vomiting.

Nausea may also result indirectly from medication prescribed by the patient's general practitioner or specialist. Though rarely two patients have the same initial symptoms, a patient who has experienced the problem of migraine for some years will know when an attack is impending. He will immediately turn to medication in an attempt to forestall the dreaded attack. The prescribed dose is rarely successful and so in his anxiety he may repeat the dosage. Too many pills may result in gastric irritation and possibly nausea and active vomiting.

Stress

It is a common belief that stress causes migraine attacks. In my opinion stress as such only occurs in the afflicted individual when the migraine attack is imminent. Stress is, in fact, one of the early **accompanying** symptoms rather than the root cause of migraine.

Stress has also been suggested as the cause of those migraine attacks that start around the time of puberty. However, this is also the time when children are expected to start prolonged studying. Thus they often spend long hours with their heads bent over their books, thus setting up all the circumstances we have described as the cause for a migraine attack. The excessive studying in preparation for an examination may equally be the cause of those attacks that occur at examination times. It may similarly be argued that although possibly the majority of migraine sufferers have above average IQ it is not this factor that causes or contributes to the onset of migraine. These patients invariably spend long hours reading, writing or painting, according to their discipline, with the head constantly held forward for long periods. This may cause constriction and then compensatory dilatation of the common carotid artery and thus set up the conditions that result in a migraine attack.

The Psychological Factor

As well as mental stress many doctors and consultants consider emotional upsets as factors in triggering migraine attacks. The early death of a parent or the untimely death of a near relative have been suggested as causes of repeated and severe attacks and the patient sent for psychiatric counselling. For patients to be referred to a psychiatrist when they are suffering from a physical problem is, in my opinion, misguided and unrewarding and may cause further considerable distress.

Hormonal Imbalance

Hormonal imbalance, I believe, has no bearing whatsoever in the migraine syndrome and certainly I have experienced no difference in the ratio of female patients to male.

As a rule, migraine sufferers have fewer and fewer attacks **after middle age.** This would seem to contradict my theory of the cause of migraine because many people in middle age develop a certain amount of fixed forward flexion of the head. However, in this age group, the arteries become slightly hardened with a loss of elasticity. Therefore, the forward flexion of the head cannot constrict the common carotid artery to the same extent and dilatation of this and other arteries does not, as a rule, occur to the same degree.

CHAPTER IV

My Treatment of Migraine

The Development of my Treatment

I HAVE explained in the Introduction how my treatment of migraine came about almost accidentally. A number of patients suffering from cervical disorders: arthritis, spondylitis or spondylosis commented on the fact that, although they were normally chronic migraine sufferers, each had not had a migraine attack after my treatment for his, or her, neck problem. I realised that within my normal treatment to the cervical area there was hidden a successful treatment, and possibly a clue to the root cause, of the migraine syndrome.

As I have explained in the previous chapter, I firmly believe the root cause of migraine is faulty posture of the head and neck. As cervical disorders, such as slipped disc lesions, spondylitis, spondylosis and arthritis all result in faulty head posture due to a lack of mobility in the neck area and consequential disuse atrophy or muscle wasting, they are perhaps worth further consideration. Most migraine sufferers show some clinical signs of these conditions or in young patients, early warnings that they may develop.

It is also interesting to note that conversely when I now ask each patient with cervical disorders if he or she suffers from headaches the answer is invariably in the affirmative. Further investigation usually shows that it is of the migraine syndrome, varying from patient to patient in its intensity.

The condition of a cervical disc lesion is quite frequently present in migraine patients and, in many cases that I see it has not previously been diagnosed. It can contribute greatly to the onset of the migraine condition and must be treated immediately before any further treatment is undertaken. The clinical signs of a cervical disc lesion

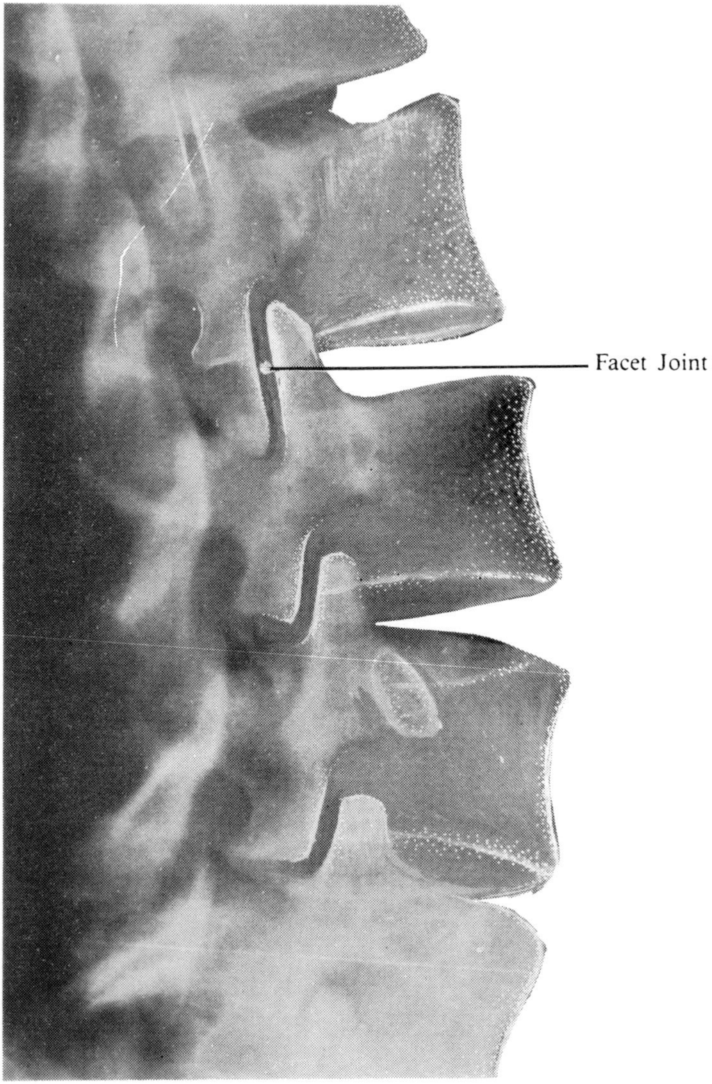

Diag. 12. Photograph of an X-ray plate showing facet joints articulating in an almost vertical plane.

have been touched on in Chapter II page 28 but a full explanation of the diagnosis and treatment of this condition is too complicated to be included here. It is however, described in great detail in my book, "The Slipped Disc and the Aching Back of Man"* The condition of a cervical slipped disc lesion, if left untreated, usually gives rise to a lateral curvature of the cervical area of the spinal column, known medically as torticollis. In this condition the head and neck are constantly held slightly forwards and to one side, setting up the conditions to produce a migraine attack.

Cervical spondylitis and spondylosis occur very frequently in patients over 40. They result in loss of cervical movement on account of the pain involved and a particular loss of side rotation of the head. This is, as a rule due to disuse atrophy of the post cervical muscles with contraction of the muscles and ligaments between opposing cervical vertebrae. The clinical signs of many migraine patients show evidence of these conditions (see Chapter II, page 28). They may show signs of the development of a "Dowager's Hump" and/or flattening of the normal cervical hollow giving rise to some fixed forward flexion of the head with rounding of the shoulders.

Cervical arthritis often causes the cartilage of the opposing surfaces of the articulating facet joints in the cervical area of the spinal column to become roughened (see diagram opposite). In some cases osteophytic outgrowths may arise. These most commonly occur on the anterior aspect of the vertebral bodies and can usually be detected by x-ray. The vertebral bodies are made up of cancellous bone, the type of bone subject to such outgrowths. The roughness of the cartilege of the affected joint surfaces is caused by the laying down of uric acid crystals on the facet joint surfaces. Any head movements, turning the head from side to side or backward rotation, will cause varying degrees of pain and audible clickings or creakings (crepitus) as the rough surfaces of the opposing arthritic facet joint surfaces rub together. It may be compared to rubbing two pieces of fine sandpaper together. If, however, the pieces of sandpaper are rubbed against one another long enough, the spikes will be rubbed smooth and no sound will be heard. Similarly, after regular exercising, the surfaces of the roughened arthritic facet joints will become smooth and polished or eburnated and the mobility of the joints will become freer and painless. Constant exercising will also help to prevent osteophytic outgrowths developing.

* 'The Slipped Disc and the Aching Back of Man' by A. Walker-Naddell published by J. R. Reid Printers Ltd. in 1985.

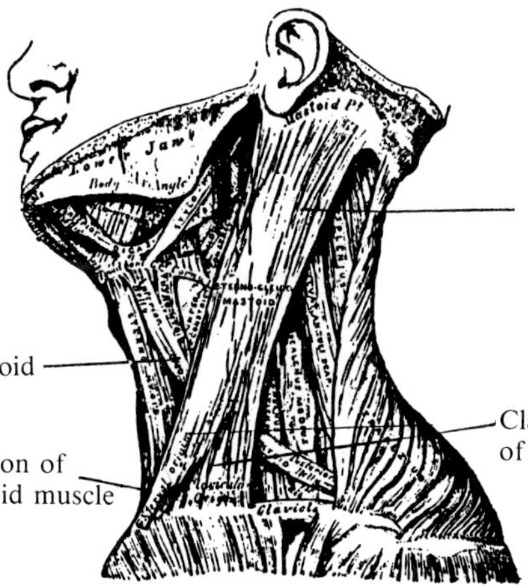

Diagram to show the sterno-mastoid and the omo-hyoid muscles.

My treatment for all these cervical disorders consists of, initially detachment of the disc if a cervical disc lesion is present, then **in all cases** 'surgical manipulation' which stretches the affected muscles and ligaments. Then the patient is given a Training Programme of four prescribed exercises which he must carry out at home. They are designed to exercise the neck muscles and joints to facilitate mobility and prevent the further laying down of uric acid crystals.

This forms the first part of my treatment for migraine to correct the faulty posture that is the underlying cause of the condition.

The four stages of 'surgical manipulation', that compare fairly closely with the four exercises of the training programme, are described carefully in the next section. They involve considerable backward extension of the head, rotation backwards of the head and side rotation of the head all performed by the consultant and finally one exercise similar to a breast stroke in swimming but this time performed by the patient, again with the head held backwards.

I realised that the backward extension that was involved in nearly all stages of the 'surgical manipulation' caused the sterno-mastoid muscles and the underlying omo-hyoid muscles to be stretched backwards, causing pressure on the dilated common carotid arteries. At the same time the artery is elongated, thus leading to a diminution of arterial blood flow to the brain. The movement of the head from side to side and when rotated backwards has a similar effect and the 'breast stroke-like' exercise causes even further stretching of the sterno-mastoid and omo-hyoid muscles. When the arms are pulled round and back with the head held right back, the sterno-mastoid omo-hyoid muscles are pulled further backwards and greater pressure is exerted on the common carotid arteries.

This slight but continued pressure exerted on the common carotid arteries, causes the dilated arteries to contract and the blood flow to the brain to become normal. This is the **'secret' of the cure for migraine.**

Very gentle and increased pressure on the dilated common carotid artery with the flat of the thumb on the affected side of the neck will similarly decrease the abnormal blood flow to the brain. The strong pulse beat will lessen after say three or four seconds. When one reaches the correct amount of blood flow to the brain by arterial pressure the higher centres in the brain will send a signal to the heart to reduce the blood flow through the common carotid artery to the normal flow. Prolonged pressure for say more than 10 seconds, on the common carotid artery, or very rapidly applied heavy pressure will result in pain and the patient becoming light-headed and dizzy. This must, of course, be avoided.

This treatment by arterial pressure is extended to all accessible arteries in the head and neck area and **forms the second and most important part of my treatment.**

In all cases I apply **very firm** pressure on the following dilated arteries of the head and neck: the posterior occipital artery, the supra and inferior orbital arteries, the temporal arteries and the facial arteries.

My Treatment of Migraine

MY TREATMENT consists of, in this order:

I. 'surgical manipulation' of the cervical area

II. treatment involving arterial pressure

III. a prescribed Training Programme of four exercises.

N.B. If a cervical disc lesion is present, this is immediately detached (see Chapter II, page 28 and also this Chapter IV, page 45).

I. The Four Stages of 'Surgical Manipulation' of the Cervical Area

All the stages in my 'surgical manipulation' have been carefully designed to increase mobility of the neck by stretching the intrinsic muscles and ligaments and smoothing the opposing facet joint surfaces at the back of the cervical column. This increased mobility will allow greater backward extension of the head and neck which in turn will produce maximum pressure by the taut sterno-mastoid and omo-hyoid muscles on the dilated common carotid arteries.

During manipulation audible clicks or creaking will be heard by myself and the patient which may be disturbing. I explain that it is merely one facet rubbing against the opposing facet on which uric acid crystals have formed. The rubbing causes the crystals to be broken off and absorbed and eventually passed out by the faecal and urinary system. This produces some freedom of movement in all the neck and supra-scapular muscles and encourages (or even allows) the patient gradually to adopt an erect posture of the head and shoulders.

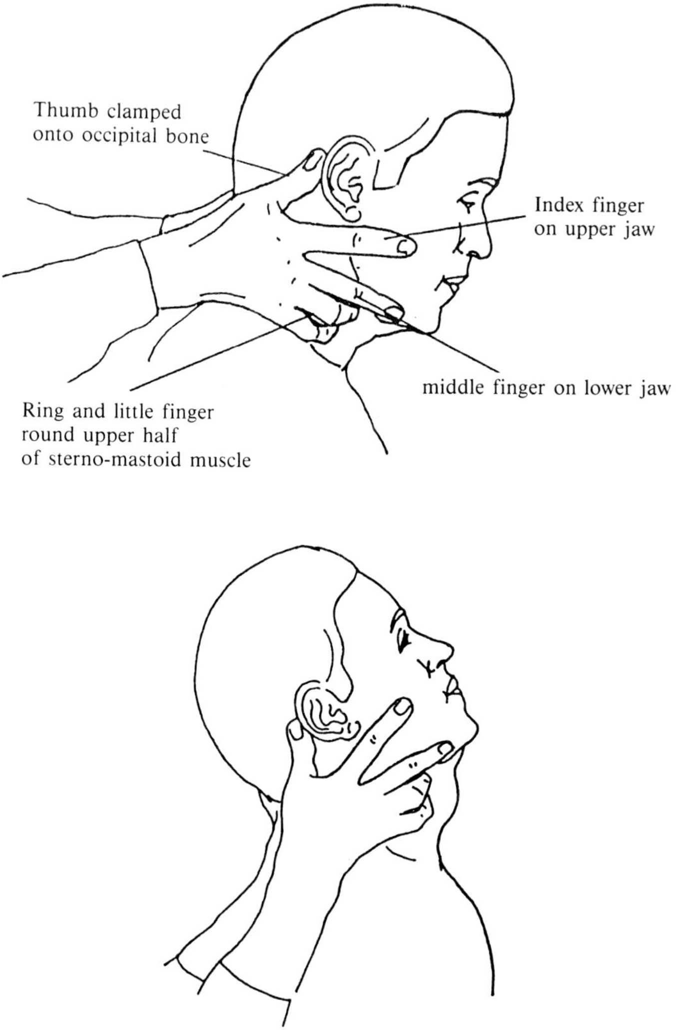

Position of hands on either side of the head during surgical manipulation of the head and neck.

During 'surgical manipulation' I prefer to have the patient standing with his back towards me. In this position I have a very firm grip of the back of the patient's head with my hands and am therefore able to carry out a full range of movements of the head and neck.

I ask the patient to take deep breaths through the nose and expire through the mouth during the manipulation.

I then place my hands firmly with outstretched fingers on either side of the back of the head and neck.

My **palms** are clamped onto either side of the skull.

My **thumbs** are pressed firmly onto the occipital bone, just behind the ears.

The **index fingers** are placed firmly along the line of the upper jaw.

The **middle fingers** are placed firmly along the lower border of the mandible.

The **ring and little fingers** are hooked into the area of the neck just in front of the upper third of the sterno-mastoid muscles, and assist in holding the whole head firmly during manipulation. Beneath these fingers i.e. the ring and little fingers the pulses of the common carotid arteries will be felt and the pulsation will be greater on the affected side.

The Walker-Naddell 'Surgical Manipulation' of the Head and Neck for Controlling Migraine

Stage I

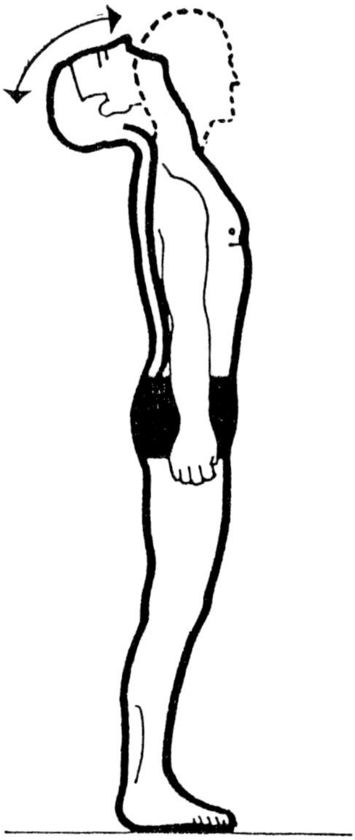

STAGE ONE OF 'SURGICAL MANIPULATION' FOR CONTROLLING MIGRAINE

I very **gently** pull the head backwards to a point just short of pain to the patient. Then I return the head to the normal erect position (never forwards) and I repeat this ten times.

In many patients with a degree of cervical spondylosis the amount of backward movement, initially will be very small indeed, but will improve fractionally after each treatment. After approximately two to three weeks the range of backward movement will be normal.

The Walker-Naddell 'Surgical Manipulation' of the Head and Neck for Controlling Migraine

Stage II

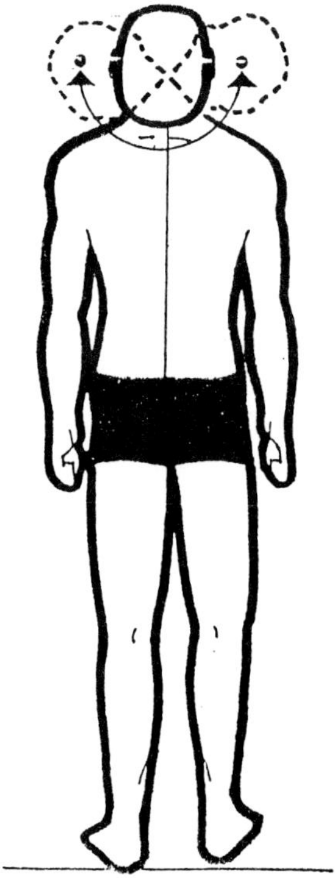

STAGE TWO OF 'SURGICAL MANIPULATION' FOR CONTROLLING MIGRAINE

With the head and neck in backward extension I hold the head very firmly between my hands and fingers; then rotate the head backwards gently to one side, the ear towards the point of the shoulder.

I return the head and neck as far as possible short of pain or discomfort along the same axis to the point of the opposite shoulder, following the course of the round part of a capital 'D'. This should be repeated five times in each direction. The head should never be rotated round and round as this will cause dizziness.

During this manoeuvre in particular the audible creakings referred to earlier will be experienced.

The Walker-Naddell 'Surgical Manipulation' of the Head and Neck for Controlling Migraine

Stage III

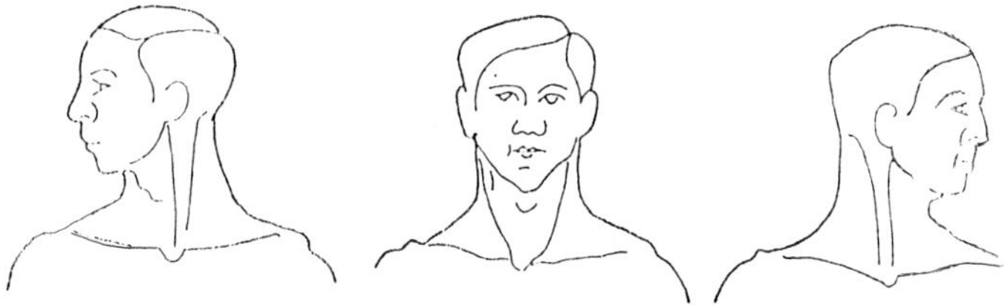

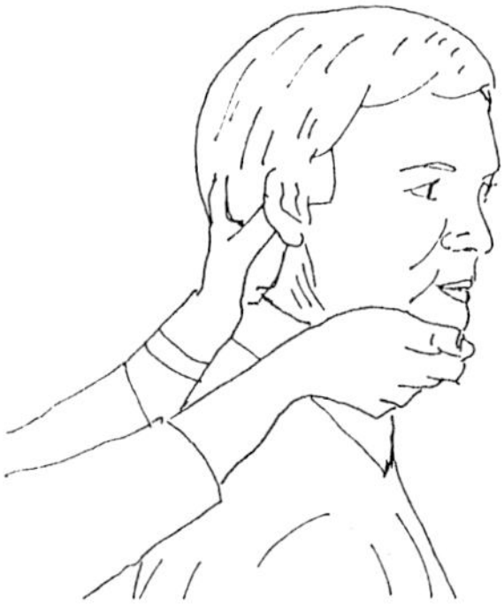

Position of hands to increase rotation of neck during Stage III.

STAGE THREE OF 'SURGICAL MANIPULATION' FOR CONTROLLING MIGRAINE

Then with the head firmly held this time erect in its normal position but tilted very slightly backwards I turn the head and neck slowly but firmly sideways, until the lower mandible is in line with the top of the shoulder or as far as possible at that consultation. I find that I invariably alter the position of my hands to increase the rotation of the head and neck (see diagram opposite). I hold for a few seconds, and then rotate the head and neck in the opposite direction, slowly.

I repeat this five times in each direction. This movement pulls the taut sterno-mastoid and omo-hyoid muscles on to the common carotid arteries.

The Walker-Naddell Surgical Manipulation of the Head and Neck (or Cervical Area) for Controlling Migraine

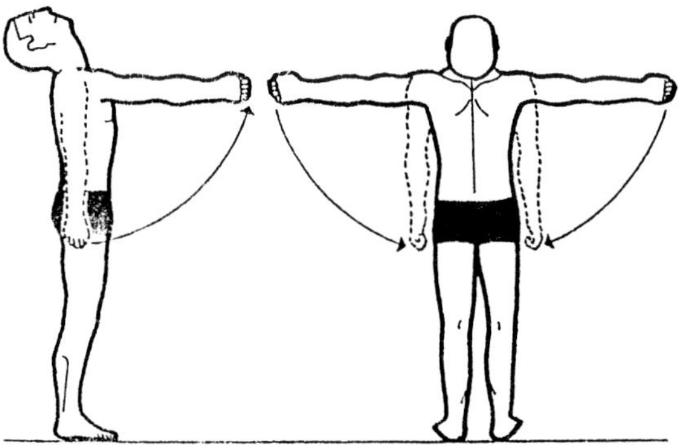

STAGE FOUR OF 'SURGICAL MANIPULATION' FOR CONTROLLING MIGRAINE

I ask the patient to perform the following exercise.

1. Stand erect with feet slightly apart.
2. Hold the head and neck back, looking up at the ceiling.
3. Stretch the arms out straight in front and parallel to the floor.
4. With the elbow joints fixed in this forward extension and fists clenched, rotate the stiff rod-like arms quickly backwards parallel to the floor until the shoulder blades meet when the arms are pulled backwards.
5. Swing the stiff arms down past the body.

I ask the patients to take a deep breath slowly through the nose when the arms are being raised to the horizontal plane, and exhale through the mouth as the shoulder blades are brought together.

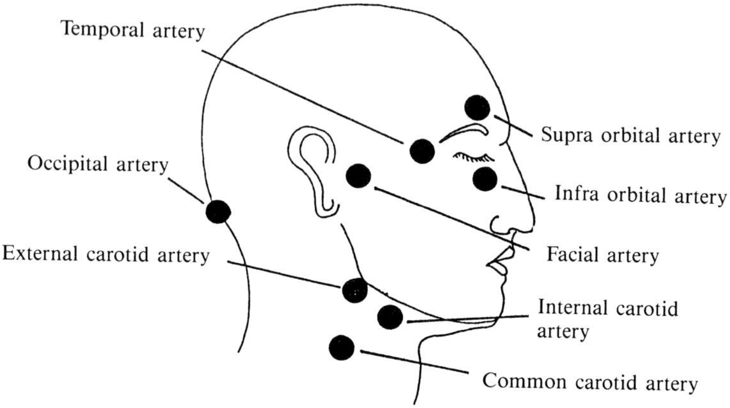

Diagram showing arterial pressure points of the neck, face and head.

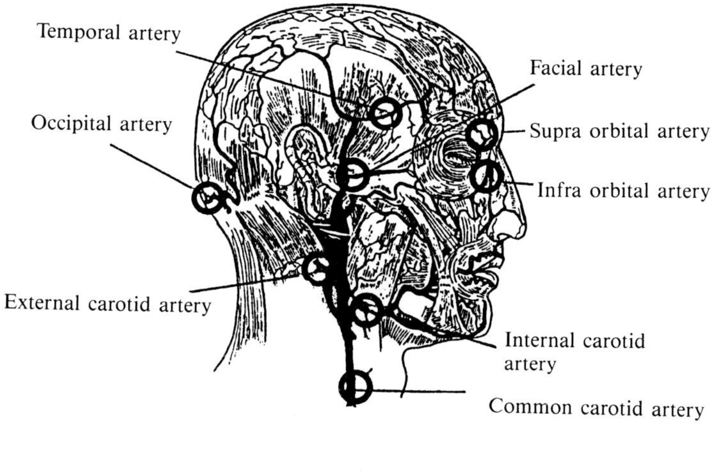

Diagram showing the superficial arteries of the neck, face and head.

II Treatment involving Arterial Pressure

1. Posterior Occipital Arteries

I apply firm pressure with my thumbs on the posterior occipital arteries at the base of the skull on either side. The head is pulled backwards to exert firmer pressure on the dilated artery, and the patient is asked to push his head backwards against my thumbs and so further increase the pressure.

2. Supra and Inferior Orbital Arteries

Similarly, I apply firm pressure with the middle fingers of both hands on the supra-orbital artery, just above the inner side of the eyebrow on both sides (more firmly on the affected side) and the inferior orbital artery just below the medial side of the eye sockets. The patient is asked to pull his head forwards to exert firmer pressure on the dilated arteries.

3. Temporal Arteries

With my middle fingers or thumbs I then compress the temporal arteries on either side of the forehead.

4. Facial Arteries

With my thumbs I compress the facial arteries on each side of the face just in front of the auricular orifices.

5. Common Carotid Arteries

In cases of **acute** migraine I examine the common carotid arteries immediately. I usually find that this large artery is dilated on one side or the other. On the affected side I very gently compress the dilated artery with the flat of my thumb, holding it in this position intially for five seconds and, in some cases, up to 10 seconds. At times, the patient will indicate that they are feeling a bit faint and, at this point, I immediately stop the light pressure. After a few minutes I am able to carry on with the same manoeuvre. This may have to be repeated three or four times, and, as a rule, it stops the migraine quite suddenly.

III The Training Programme

This is so important that for the convenience of reference I have allocated it a complete chapter (see page 65).

At the end of the consultation the patient is counselled to avoid long periods of holding the head in forward flexion, to take regular breaks from such a posture. He is advised that the onset of a migraine attack can often be prevented by adopting a different sleeping position: that is by arranging his pillows so that his head will not fall forwards or laterally and thus remain in forward flexion during the long hours of sleep. He must carry out the training programme of four exercises assiduously and consistently at least four times every day and more frequently if possible. I always stress the value of breathing properly during this Training programme.

CHAPTER V

The Training Programme of Four Exercises to Avoid Migraine

BECAUSE migraine is caused by faulty, and often fixed, forward posture of the head that is commonly the result of the patient holding his head forward for prolonged periods, I prescribe the following programme of exercises, that are designed primarily to tone the neck and supra-scapular muscles in order to support the head in its correct alignment. Regular exercising will also restore mobility of the joints affected by osteo-arthritis by smoothing the roughened surfaces of the opposing facet joints of the cervical area of the spinal column.

The exercises should be done initially as often as is practicable, at least four times a day, but I also recommend to my patients that they carry out this training programme for a minute or two, night and morning, **for all time.**

However, if the patient feels an attack coming on, he should immediately stop whatever he may be doing and at once carry out the full training programme, sitting in an upright chair. This will stop the impending attack right away.

On average, it usually takes 2-3 weeks for the condition to resolve and a full range of movement to be obtained. Patients are advised to carry out all the movements of the exercises very gently, especially at first. They should avoid causing the slightest pain whilst exercising, because this would retard progress in the training. This applies to all training regardless of the areas which are being exercised. There is in time, practically no pain with a normal range of movements. The patient should be warned however that on the day following the commencement of treatment, there will be some muscle ache, similar to that which occurs when one has played the first game of sport at the beginning of the season. This aching is simply the start of the muscles coming into action after a disuse atrophy. It should settle after two or three days, and more and more freedom of movement with less and less discomfort will be achieved.

Breathing

Deep breaths must be taken throughout the exercising, for breathing is a very important factor in any type of exercise or training. Patients are advised to draw air in through the nose and exhale by the mouth. Inhalation through the nose enables deeper breaths to be taken which fill the lungs and thereby immediately feeds oxygen to all muscles which are in use, and, in fact to every part of the body. The oxygen is extracted from the air and carried by the red blood cells in the arterial blood stream to all parts of the body. Without oxygen muscles will not regenerate and the patient will tire very quickly. Normal exhalation by mouth dispels the products of muscle usage i.e. carbon dioxide and lactic acid.

Deep breathing also causes the chest to expand. The head is gently thrown backwards; rounding of the dorsal spine is partially flattened and the normal lumbar lordosis marginally increased, giving rise to a better posture.

For all the four exercises the patient may stand or sit. When sitting the patient should use a dining chair, without arms, the back of which should only come up to shoulder level. He should sit well back into the chair so that his lumbar and dorsal areas of the spinal column are well supported. This prevents strain in the lumbar area if the patient has any lower back trouble but allows free movement of the neck and shoulder joints. In fact the **advantage of sitting** to perform the exercises is that it concentrates all the movement in the neck and shoulder areas for which the exercises were primarily designed.

At the first appointment the four exercises are executed under my close scrutiny to make sure they are done absolutely correctly in the exact sequence 1, 2, 3, 4 to my complete satisfaction.

THE FUNCTIONS OF THE TRAINING PROGRAMME

The main aims of the Training Programme may be summarised as follows:

1. They have been designed to tone the muscles at the back of the neck.
2. They also stretch the skin and unyielding underlying fascia at the front of the neck, pulling the muscles at the front of the neck, the sterno-mastoid and omo-hyoid muscles on to the dilated common carotid arteries.
3. They stretch the intrinsic muscles and ligaments of the whole cervical region.
4. They improve mobility of the cervical joints by smoothing the opposing rough surfaces of the facet joints.

The Walker-Naddell Training Programme for Controlling Migraine

Exercise I

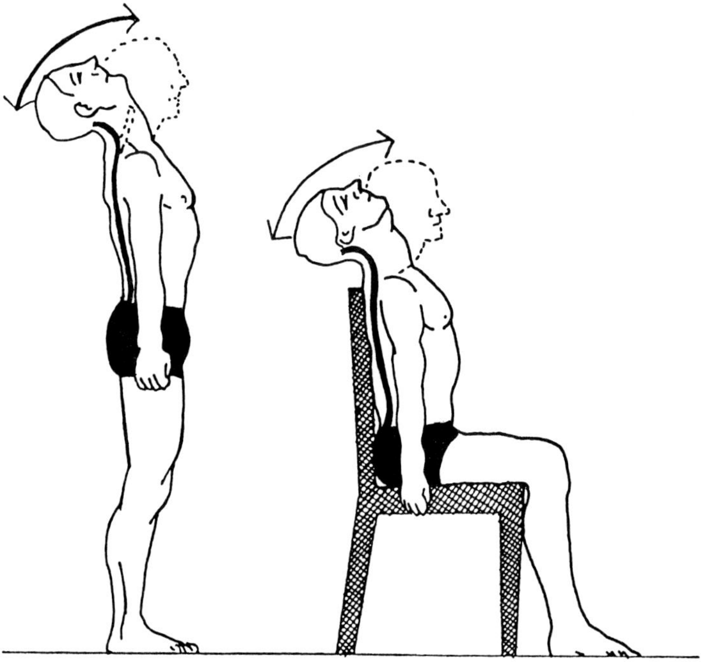

The Walker-Naddell Training Programme for Controlling Migraine

Exercise I

1. Draw the head backwards very gently until stiffness occurs and pain presents itself. Then return the head forwards but only as far as the erect posture, (never bending the neck forwards).
2. Repeat 10 times.

The Walker-Naddell Training Programme for Controlling Migraine

Exercise II

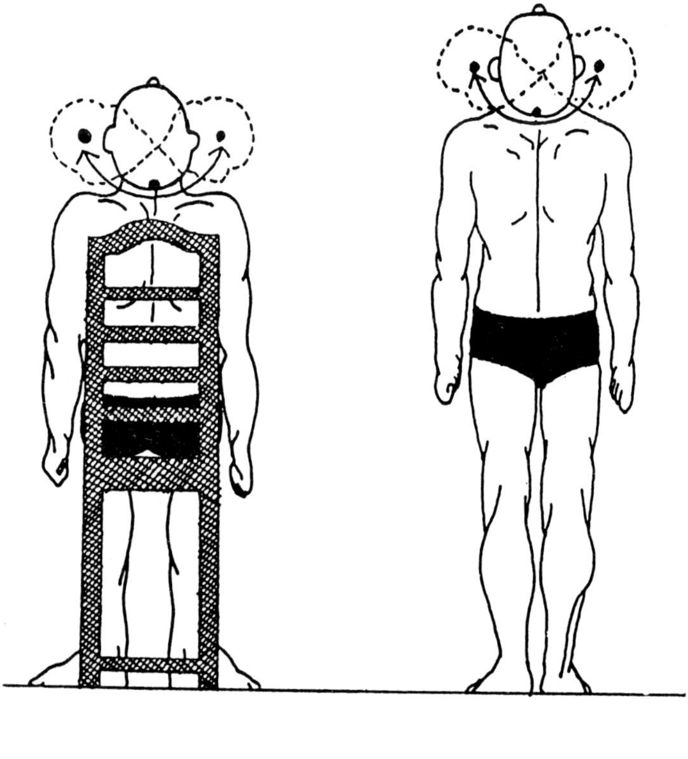

The Walker-Naddell Training Programme for Controlling Migraine

Exercise II

1. Hold the head backwards.
2. Rotate the head in this axis, ear to shoulder, five times to one side. Avoid bringing the head forwards beyond the shoulder point.
3. Similarly, rotate in the opposite direction five times.
4. The rotation should follow the course of the round part of a capital 'D'.

N.B. The head should never be rotated round and round as this will cause dizziness.

The Walker-Naddell Training Programme for Controlling Migraine

Exercise III

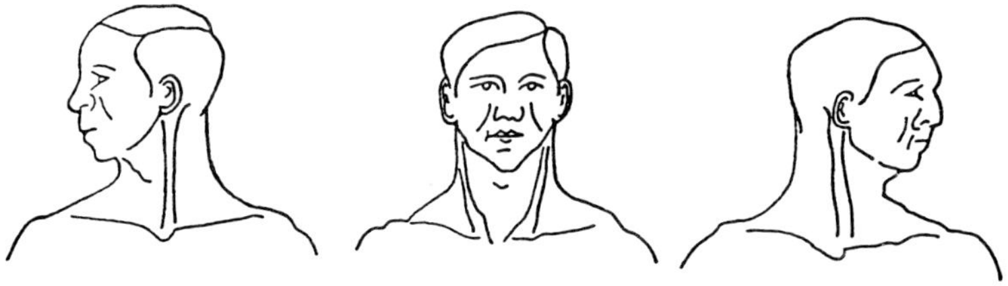

A

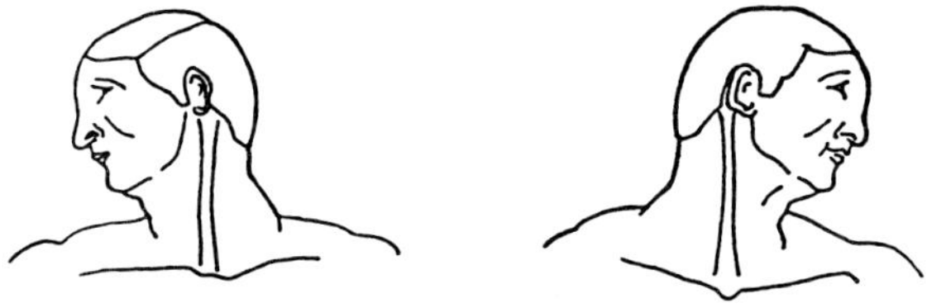

B

In B head is tilted backwards to increase pressure by muscles on structures underlying them.

The Walker-Naddell Training Programme for Controlling Migraine

Exercise III

1. With the head erect and tilted slightly backwards, turn the neck slowly but firmly sideways, until the chin as far as possible is in line with the top of the shoulder.
   Then pause for a count of three.

2. Perform the exercise five times in each direction, three or four times a day.

The Walker-Naddell Training Programme for Controlling Migraine

Exercise IV

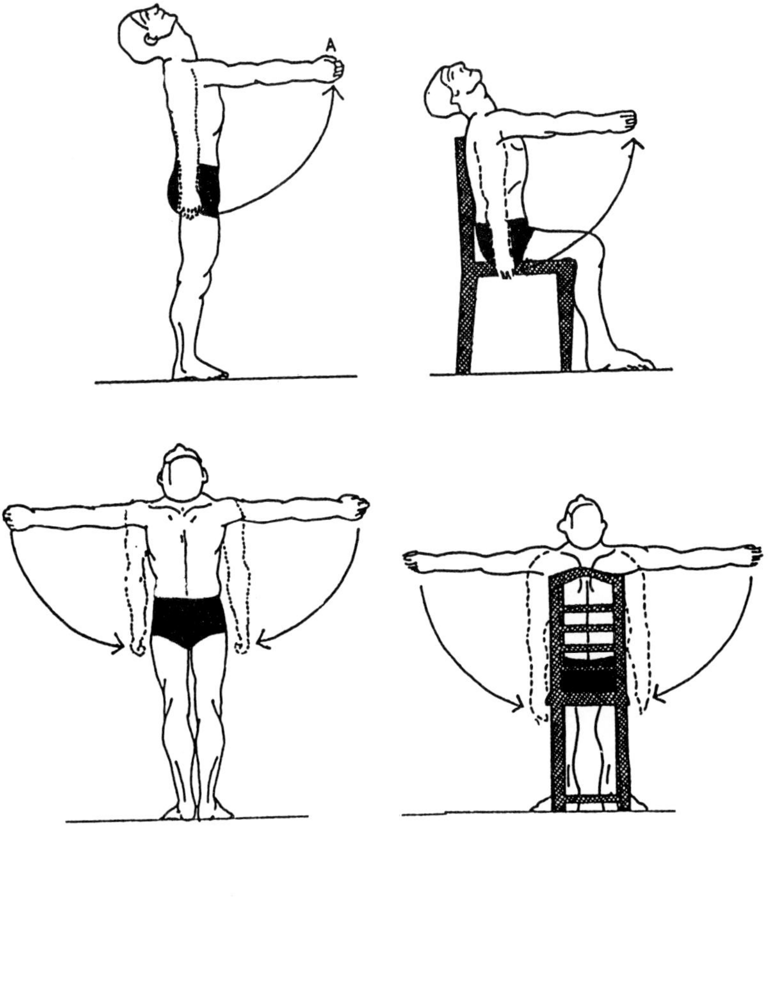

The Walker-Naddell Training Programme for Controlling Migraine

Exercise IV

1. Hold the head back, looking up to the ceiling.
2. Keep the arms taut, like rods.
3. Stretch the arms out straight in front and parallel to the floor.
4. With elbow joints fixed and fists clenched, rotate the stiff arms quickly backwards with the shoulder blades coming together when the rod-like arms are right back.
5. Swing the stiff arms down past the body and repeat 10 times, four times a day.

Take a deep breath through the nose when the arms are being raised to the horizontal plane, and exhale as the shoulder blades are brought together and the arms are lowered to the side of the body.

During this exercise the omo-hyoid muscle, which is attached to the scapular and the hyoid bone, is stretched like a cord over the dilated common carotid artery, thus assisting the contraction of the artery, and diminishing the blood flow to the brain, head and neck.

This exercise not only tones the muscles of the neck but also the supra-scapular, medial scapular and the arm muscles. If there is a degree of cervical spondylosis present, exercies II and IV — the rotation of the head in the shape of a 'D' and the above exercise — will tone up the affected muscles and a full range of movement will in time be obtained.

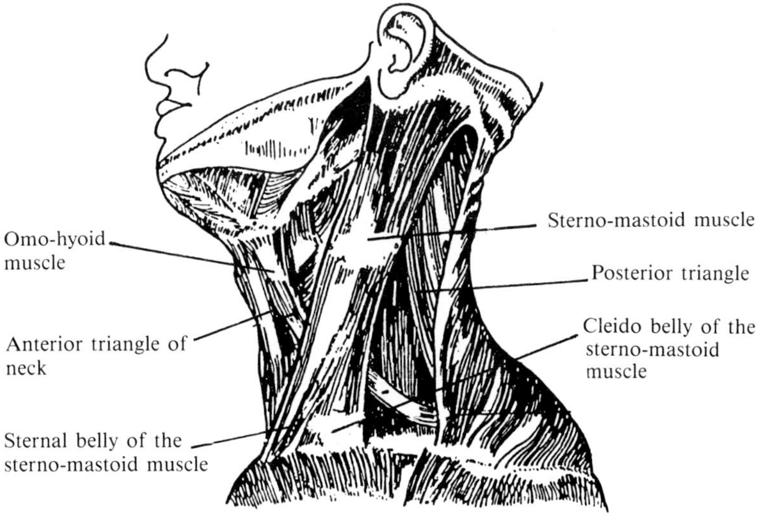

Diagram to show the sterno-mastoid and the omo-hyoid muscles and the two triangles of the neck.

APPENDIX A

SOME notes on the anatomy of the Head and Neck in so far as they are relevant to the study of Migraine.

This anatomy section is based on Gray's Anatomy, the definitive work on anatomy and the physicians' 'Bible'!

The Triangles of the Neck

The anatomy of the large arteries of the neck and their branches and the relations they bear to the veins and nerves, should be examined collectively as they present themselves in certain regions of the neck.

The side of the neck presents a somewhat quadrilateral outline, limited above, by the lower border of the body of the jaw, and an imaginary line extending from the angle of the jaw to the mastoid process; below, by the prominent upper border of the clavicle; in front, by the median line of the neck; behind, by the anterior margin of the Trapezius muscle. This space is subdivided into two large triangles by the Sterno-mastoid muscle, which passes obliquely across the neck, from the sternum and clavicle below, to the mastoid process above. The triangular space in front of this muscle is called the anterior triangle and that behind it, the posterior angle. These two large triangles at the side of the neck are subdivided into two smaller triangles by the omo-hyoid muscle.

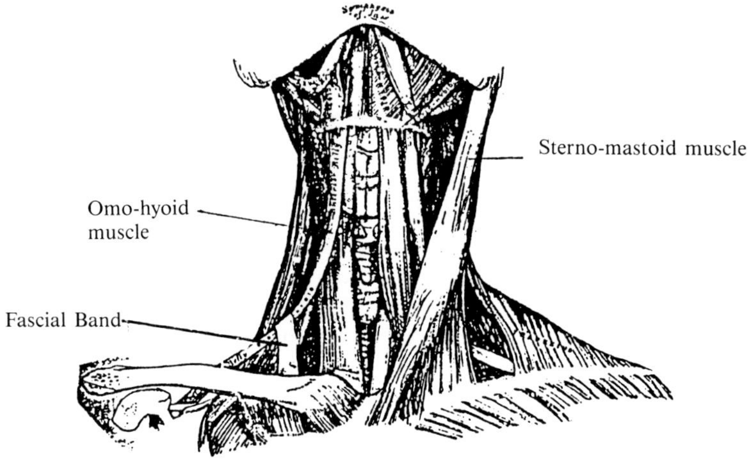

Diagram to show the omo-hyoid muscle, the sterno-mastoid muscle and the fascia.

The Omo-Hyoid Muscle

This is so important to my thesis on migraine that it deserves detailed attention. It lies immediately behind the lower third of the sterno-mastoid muscle and transverses over the fibrous sheath containing the common carotid artery, the pneumogastric nerve and the internal jugular vein.

The Omo-hyoid passes across the side of the neck, from the scapula to the hyoid bone. It may be considered as made up of two muscular sections, united by a central tendon. It arises from the upper border of the scapula, and crosses the suprascapular notch. Its extent of attachment to the scapula is usually one inch. From this origin, the posterior muscular section inclines forward and slightly upwards across the lower part of the neck behind the Sterno-mastoid muscle, where it becomes tendinous and, passing in front of the fibrous tube which contains the common carotid artery, the jugular vein and the pneumogastric nerve, it then changes direction forming an obtuse angle and terminates in the anterior muscular section, which passes almost vertically upwards, to be inserted into the lower border of the body of the hyoid bone. The central tendon of this muscle, which varies much in length and form is held in position by a process of deep cervical fascia, which includes it in a sheath. This process is prolonged down, to be attached to the clavicle and first rib. It is by this means that the angular form of the muscle is maintained.

RELATIONS: By its superficial surface, with the Trapezius, the Sterno-mastoid, deep cervical fascia, Platysma, and skin. By its deep surface, with the Scaleni muscles, phrenic nerve, lower cervical nerves, which go to form the brachial plexus, the suprascapular vessels and nerve, deep unyielding cervical sheath of fascia, enclosing the common carotid artery, the pneumogastric nerve and the internal jugular vein.

ACTIONS: These muscles depress the larynx and hyoid bone, after they have been drawn up with the pharynx in the act of swallowing. The Omo-hyoid muscles not only depress the hyoid bone, but carry it backwards, and to one or the other side. It is concerned specially in prolonged inspiratory efforts; for by tensing the lower part of the cervical fascia it lessens the inward suction of the soft parts, which would otherwise compress the great vessels of the neck i.e. the common carotid artery, the internal jugular vein and the pneumogastric nerve and the apices of the lungs.

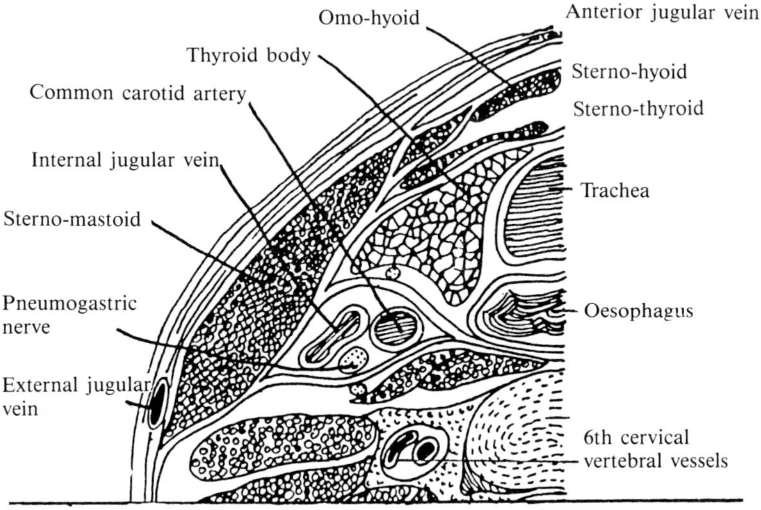

Section of the neck at about the level of the sixth cervical vertebra, showing the arrangement of the deep cervical fascia.

The central tendon of the omo-hyoid muscle is of vital importance as a factor in the cause of the migraine syndrome. When the head is in forward flexion for prolonged periods this central tendon exerts mechanical pressure on first the internal jugular vein as it is placed anterior to the artery and nerve. This may lead to slight cerebral congestion. Mechanical pressure is then progressively exerted on the common carotid artery. This will initially cause stricture of the artery. From this follows the dilatation of the arteries to combat the mild ischaemia to the brain and results in the symptoms of the migraine syndrome (see Chapter III page 35).

There is considerable variation in the length and size of the central tendon. At times the tendon is found to be rather large and the fascia which holds it down to the clavicle and first rib is short. In these circumstances movement of the neck may cause over-stretching of the omo-hyoid muscle and this may produce a greater tendency for migraine to occur.

The treatment of migraine is primarily concerned with the anatomy and function of three different structures: arteries, nerves and veins and thus this chapter will describe and illustrate in turn:

The arteries of the head and neck

The nerves of the head and neck

The veins of the head and neck

in so far as these are relevant to the migraine syndrome.

The Arteries of the Head and Neck

Arteries are cylindrical, tubular vessels that convey the blood from both ventricles of the heart to every part of the body. They are dense in structure, very strong and highly elastic. Arteries may subdivide either into two equal branches or several smaller branches. Arteries communicate with each other through anastomoses which occur when great activity of circulation is required, as in the brain. The larger arterial branches in the body follow a comparatively straight course but in some situations arteries pursue a more tortuous route. This is the case with the facial artery in its course over the face and with the internal carotid before it enters the cavity of the skull. These curves in the arteries serve to diminish the velocity of the current of blood by increasing the extent of surface over which the arteries move.

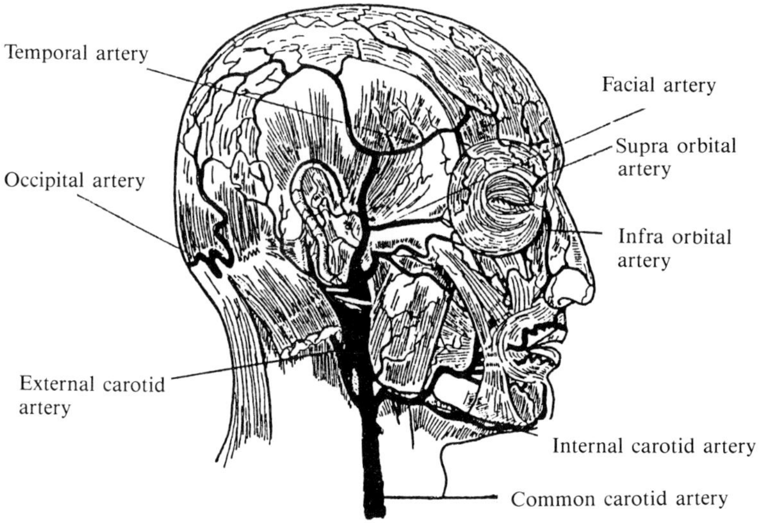

Diagram showing the superficial arteries of the neck, face and head.

The Common Carotid Artery plays an important part in the study and treatment of migraine. It is the major artery that supplies the head and neck with blood from the heart. It ascends in the neck and divides into two branches: the **External Carotid,** supplying the superficial parts of the head and face and the greater part of the neck; and the **Internal Carotid,** supplying the internal parts of the cranium and orbit.

Despite the differences of origin in the neck, the right and left common carotids resemble each other so closely, that one description will apply to both. Each vessel passes obliquely upwards, from behind the sterno-clavicular articulation, to a level with the upper border of the thyroid cartilage, opposite the fourth cervical vertebra, where it divides into the external and internal carotids.

At the lower part of the neck the two common carotid arteries are separated from each other by a very small interval, which contains the trachea; but at the upper part, the thyroid body, the larynx and pharynx project forwards between the two vessels, and give the appearance of their being placed farther back in this situation. The **common carotid artery** is contained in a sheath derived from the deep cervical fascia, which also encloses **the internal jugular vein and pneumogastric nerve,** the vein lying on the outer side of the artery, and the nerve between the artery and vein, on a plane posterior to both. On opening the sheath, these three structures are seen to be separated from one another, each being enclosed in a separate fibrous investment.

The carotid arteries are covered throughout their entire extent by the sterno-mastoid muscle, but their course does not correspond to the anterior border of the muscle, which passes somewhat in a curved direction from the mastoid process to the sterno-clavicular joint. The course of the artery is indicated more exactly by a line drawn from the sternal end of the clavicle below, to a point midway between the angle of the jaw and the mastoid process above. The portion of line below the level of the upper border of the thyroid cartilage would represent the course of the vessel.

The common carotid arteries may be compressed to control dilatation by firmly applying pressure with the fingers or thumbs on either side of the neck, slightly displacing the sterno-mastoid muscle.

I. **The External Carotid Artery** commences opposite the upper border of the thyroid cartilage, and, taking a slightly curved course, passes upwards and forwards, and then inclines backwards to the space between the neck of the condyle of the lower jaw and the external meatus, where it divides into the temporal and internal maxillary arteries. It rapidly diminishes in size in its course up the neck, owing to the number and large size of the branches given off from it. In the child, it is somewhat smaller than the internal carotid; but in the adult, the two vessels are of nearly equal size. At its commencement, this artery is more superficial, and placed nearer the middle line than the internal carotid.

The external carotid artery gives off eight branches. Of these four are of major importance in the treatment of migraine. These only will be considered in detail viz:

1. The facial artery
2. The occipital artery
3. The superficial temporal artery
4. The internal maxillary, in particular the infra-orbital artery

1. The Facial Artery

In the neck, its origin is superficial, being covered by the integument, platysma muscle and fascia. On the face, where it passes over the body of the lower jaw, it is comparatively superficial, lying immediately beneath the platysma. In this situation its pulsation may be distinctly felt, and compression of the vessel against the bone can be effectively made to control dilatation. The facial vein lies to the outer side of the artery, and takes a more direct course across the face, where it is separated from the artery by a considerable interval. In the neck it lies superficial to the artery. The branches of the facial nerve cross the artery and the infra-orbital nerve lies beneath it.

2. **The Post-occipital Artery.** The post-occipital artery arises from the posterior part of the external carotid, opposite the facial, near the lower margin of the Digastric muscle. At its origin, it is covered by the posterior belly of the Digastric and stylo-hyoid muscles, and the hypoglossal nerve winds around it from behind forwards: higher up, it passes across the internal carotid artery, the internal jugular vein, and the pneumogastric and spinal accessory nerves; it then ascends to the interval between the transverse process of the atlas and the mastoid process of the temporal bone, and passes horizontally backwards, grooving the surface of the latter bone. It then changes its course and passes vertically upwards, pierces the fascia which connects the cranial attachment of the trapezius with the sterno-

mastoid, and ascends in a tortuous course over the occiput, as high as the vertex, where it divides into numerous branches. It is accompanied in the latter part of its course by the great occipital, and occasionally by a cutaneous filament from the sub-occipital nerve.

3. **The Superficial Temporal Artery,** the smaller of the two terminal branches of the external carotid, appears, from its direction, to be the continuation of that vessel. It commences in the interspace between the neck of the lower jaw and the external auditory meatus, and divides into two branches, an anterior and a posterior.

3a. **The Anterior Temporal** runs tortuously upwards and forwards to the forehead, supplying the muscles, integument (the skin) and pericranium (outer surface of the skull) in this region, and anastomoses with the supra-orbital and frontal arteries.

3b. **The Posterior Temporal,** larger than the anterior, curves upwards and backwards along the side of the head, lying superficial to the temporal fascia, and joins with its fellow of the opposite side, and with the posterior auricular and occipital branches.

The superficial temporal artery is covered by a dense fascia given off from the parotid gland: it is crossed by the temporo-facial division of the facial nerve and one or two veins, and is accompanied by the **auriculo-temporal** nerve, which lies behind it.

4. **The Infra-orbital Artery.** The internal maxillary is the larger of the two terminal branches of the external carotid and the infra-orbital appears, from its direction, to be the continuation of the trunk of the internal maxillary. It often arises from that vessel by a common trunk with the preceding branch, and runs along the infra-orbital canal with the **superior maxillary nerve,** emerging upon the face at the infra-orbital foramen, beneath the Levator labii superioris. While contained in the canal, it gives off branches which ascend into the orbit, and assist in supplying the inferior rectus and inferior oblique muscles behind the eye and the lachrymal gland or tear gland. Other

branches (anterior dental) descend through the anterior dental canals in the bone, to supply the mucous membrane of the antrum, and the front teeth of the upper jaw. On the face, some branches pass upwards to the inner angle of the orbit and the lachrymal sac, anastomosing with the angular branch of the facial artery; other branches pass inwards towards the nose, anastomosing with the nasal branch of the ophthalmic; and other branches descend beneath the Lavator labii superioris, (upper lip) and anastomose with the transverse facial and buccal arteries inside the cheek.

II **The Internal Carotid Artery**

The internal carotid artery supplies the anterior part of the brain, the eye and its appendages, and sends branches to the forehead and nose. Its size, in the adult, is equal to that of the external carotid, though, in the child, it is larger than that vessel. It is remarkable for the number of curvatures that it presents in different parts of its course. It occasionally has one or two flexures near the base of the skull, while in its passage through the carotid canal and along the side of the body of the sphenoid bone it describes a double curvature which resembles the italic letter 's' placed horizontally. These curvatures most probably diminish the velocity of the current of blood, by increasing the extent of surface over which it moves, and adding to the amount of impediment produced from friction.

In considering the course and relations of this vessel, it may be conveniently divided into four portions: cervical, petrous, cavernous, and cerebral. Of these, two only are relevant in the treatment of migraine: a) cervical and b) cavernous.

IIa **The Cervical Portion of the Internal Carotid**

This portion of the internal carotid commences at the bifurcation of the common carotid, opposite the upper border of the thyroid cartilage, and runs perpendicularly upwards, in front of the transverse processes of the three upper cervical vertebrae, to the carotid canal in the petrous portion of the temporal bone. It is superficial at its commencement, being contained in the superior carotid triangle, and lying on the same level as the external carotid, but behind that artery, overlapped by the Sterno-mastoid, and covered by the deep fascia, platysma, and skin: it then passes beneath the parotid gland, being crossed by the hypoglossal nerve, the Digastric and Stylo-hyoid muscles, and the occipital and posterior auricular arteries. Higher up, it is separated from the external carotid by the Stylo-glossus and the Stylo-pharyngeus muscles, the glosso-pharyngeal nerve, and the pharyngeal branch of the pneumogastric. It is in relation, behind, with the Rectus capitis anticus major, the superior cervical ganglion of the sympathetic, and superior laryngeal nerve; externally, with the internal jugular vein and pneumogastric nerve, the nerve lying on a plane posterior to the artery; internally, with the pharynx, tonsil, the superior laryngeal nerve, and ascending pharyngeal artery. **At the base of the skull the glosso-pharyngeal, pneumogastric or vagus, spinal accessory, and hypoglossal nerves lie between the artery and the internal jugular vein.**

IIb The Cavernous Portion of the Internal Carotid Artery

The **ophthalmic artery** is one of the branches given off from the cavernous portion of the internal carotid. The branches of this vessel may be divided into an orbital group which are distributed to the orbit and surrounding parts and an ocular group which supplies the muscles and globe of the eye. Of these the supra-orbital artery deserves further description in relation to the treatment of migraine.

The Supra-Orbital Artery

The supra-orbital artery arises from the ophthalmic as that vessel is crossing over the optic nerve. Ascending so as to rise above all the muscles of the orbit, **it runs forwards, with the supra-orbital nerve,** between the periosteum and Levator palpebrae: and, passing through the supra-orbital foramen, divides into a superficial and a deep branch, which supply the integument or skin, the muscles, and the pericranium of the forehead, anastomosing with the frontal, the anterior branch of the temporal, and the artery of the opposite side. This artery in the orbit supplies the superior rectus and the Levator palpebrae, and sends a branch inwards, across the pulley of the superior oblique muscle, to supply the parts at the inner canthus of the eye. At the supra-orbital foramen it frequently transmits a branch to the diploe.

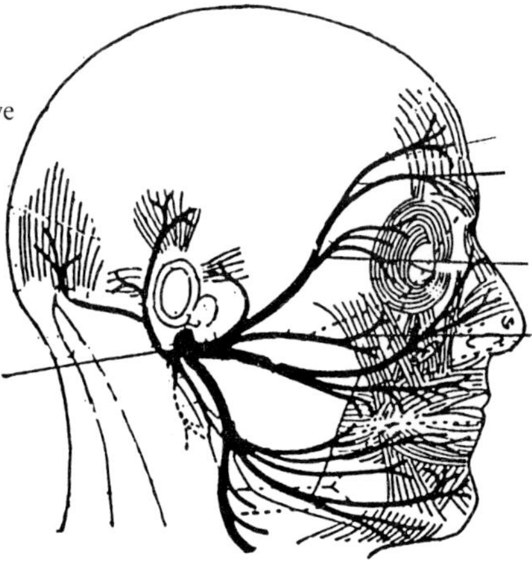

Diagram showing the relative positions of the important nerves of the head.

The Nerves of the Head and Neck
(Relevant to the Treatment of Migraine)

THE nervous tissues of the body are composed in **two great systems — the cerebro-spinal and the sympathetic** and each of these systems consists of a central organ, or series of central organs, and of nerves.

The cerebro-spinal system comprises the brain (including the medulla oblongata), the spinal cord, the cranial nerves, the spinal nerves, and the ganglia connected with both these classes of nerves. The sympathetic system consists of a double chain of ganglia, with the nerves which go to and come from them. It is not directly connected with the brain or spinal cord, though it is so indirectly by means of its numerous communications with the cranial and spinal nerves.

All these nervous tissues are composed chiefly of two different structures — the grey and the white or fibrous. It is in the former, as is generally supposed, that nervous impressions and impulses originate, and by the latter that they are conducted. Hence the grey matter forms the essential constituent of all the ganglionic centres, both those in the isolated ganglia and those aggregated in the cerebro-spinal axis; while the white matter is found in all the commissural portions of the nerve-centres and in all the cerebro-spinal nerves.

The Cranial Nerves

The cranial nerves arise from some part of the cerebrospinal

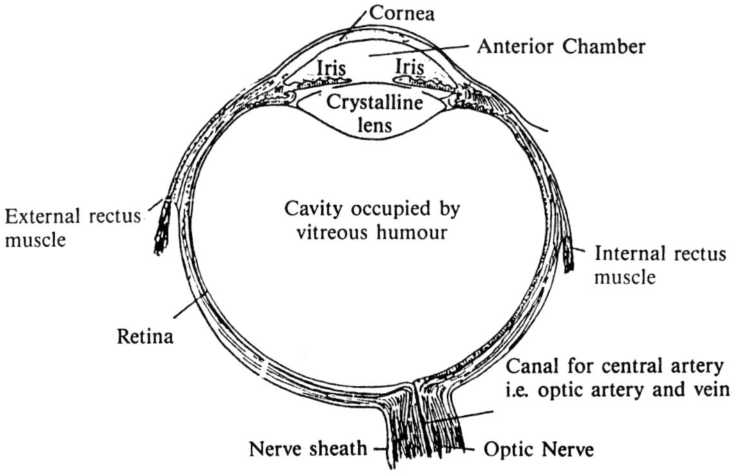

A horizontal section of the eyeball.

centre, and are transmitted through foramina in the base of the cranium. They have been named numerically, according to the order in which they pass through the dura mater lining the base of the skull. Other names are also given to them, derived from the parts to which they are distributed or from their functions. Taken in their order, from before backward, they are as follows:

1. Olfactory
2. Optic
3. Motor oculi
4. Trochlear
5. Trifacial
6. Abducent
7. Facial
8. Auditory
9. Glosso-pharyngeal
10. Pneumogastric (or Vagus)
11. Spinal Accessory
12. Hypoglossal

The **first cranial** or the **Olfactory nerves,** the special nerves of the sense or smell, are about 20 in number.

The **second** or **Optic nerve,** the special nerve of the sense of sight, is distributed exclusively to the eyeball. The nerves of opposite sides are connected together at the commissure, and from the back of the commissure they may be traced to the brain, under the name of the optic tracts.

The optic nerves arise from the fore part of the commissure.

The nerve passes forward and outward through the cavity of the orbit, pierces the sclerotic and choroid coats at the back part of the eyeball, about one-eighth of an inch to the nasal side of its centre and expands into the retina. A small artery, the **central retinal artery,** perforates the **optic nerve** a little behind the globe, and runs along its interior in a tubular canal of fibrous tissue. It supplies the inner surface of the retina, and is accompanied by corresponding **veins.**

The third or **motor oculi nerve** supplies all the muscles of the orbit except the Superior oblique and External rectus; it also supplies, through its connection with the ciliary ganglion, the Sphincter muscle of the iris and the Ciliary muscle. It is rather a large nerve, of rounded form and firm texture.

On emerging from the brain, the nerve is invested with a sheath of pia mater, and enclosed in a prolongation from the arachnoid.

The **fourth or trochlear nerve,** the smallest of the cranial nerves, supplies the Superior oblique muscle, which controls the ability to turn the eye downward and outward.

The **fifth or Trifacial nerve** is the largest cranial nerve. It resembles a spinal nerve (1) in arising by two roots; (2) in having a ganglion developed on its posterior root; and (3) in its function, since it is a compound nerve. It is the great sensory nerve of the head and face and the motor nerve of the muscles of mastication. Its upper two divisions are entirely sensory; the third division is partly sensory and partly motor. It arises by two roots: of these the anterior is the smaller, and is the motor root; the posterior, the larger and the sensory.

The two roots of the nerve pass forward below the tentorium cerebelli at its bridges over the notch on the inner part of the superior border of the petrous portion of the temporal bone: they then run between the bone and the dura mater to the apex of the petrous portion of the temporal bone, where the fibres of the sensory root form a large semilunar ganglion.

From its anterior border of the ganglion, which is directed forward and outward, three large branches proceed — the ophthalmic, superior maxillary and inferior maxillary.

1. The **ophthalmic nerve** or first division of the fifth, is a sensory nerve. It supplies the eyeball, the lachrymal gland, the mucous lining of the eye and nasal fossae, and the integument or skin of the eyebrow, forehead and nose.

Just before entering the orbit, through the sphenoidal fissure it divides into three branches — a) lachrymal, b) frontal and c) nasal.

a) The **lachrymal** is the smallest of the three branches of the ophthalmic. It sometimes receives a filament from the fourth nerve but this is possibly derived from the branch of communication which passes from the ophthalmic to the fourth. It passes forward in a separate tube of dura mater, and enters the orbit through **the narrowest part of the sphenoidal fissure.** In the orbit it runs along the upper border of the External rectus muscle, with the **lachrymal artery,** and communicates with the tempero-malar branch of the superior maxillary. It enters the lachrymal gland and gives off several filaments, which supply the gland and the conjunctiva. Finally, it pierces the superior palpebral ligament, and terminates in the integument of the upper eyelid, joining with filaments of the facial nerve.

b) The **frontal** is the largest division of the ophthalmic, and may be regarded, both from its size and direction, as the continuation of the nerve. It enters the orbit above the muscles, through the sphenoidal fissure, and runs forward along the middle line, between the Levator palpebrae and the periosteum. Midway between the apex and the base of the orbit it divides into two branches, **supratrochlear** and **supra-orbital.**

The supratrochlear branch, the smaller of the two, passes inward, above the pulley of the superior oblique muscle, and gives off a descending filament, which joins with the infratrochlear branch of the nasal nerve. It then escapes from the orbit between the pulley of the Superior oblique and supra-orbital foramen, curves up on to the forehead close to the bone, and supplies the muscles around the orbit, the Occipito-frontalis muscles, and, dividing into branches which pierce these muscles, it supplies the integument of the lower part of the forehead on either side of the middle line and sends filaments to the conjunctiva and skin of the upper lid.

The supra-orbital branch passes forward through the supra-orbital foramen, and gives off, in this situation, palpebral filaments to the upper eyelid. It then ascends upon the forehead, and terminates in cutaneous and pericranial branches. The cutaneous branches, two in number, an inner and an outer, supply the integument of the cranium as far back as the occiput. They are at first situated beneath the Occipito-frontalis, the inner branch perforating the frontal portion of the muscle, the outer branch its tendinous aponeurosis. The pericranial branches are distributed to the pericranium over the frontal and parietal bones.

c) The **nasal nerve** is intermediate in size between the frontal and lachrymal, and more deeply placed than the other branches of the ophthalmic. It enters the orbit between the two heads of the External rectus, and passes obliquely inward across the optic nerve, to the inner wall of the orbit, cranium, on the front of the cribriform plate of the ethmoid bone, through a slit into the nose, where it divides into two branches, an internal and an external.

2. **The Superior Maxillary,** or second divisiion of the fifth, is a sensory nerve. It is intermediate both in position and size, between the ophthalmic and inferior maxillary. It then crosses the spheno-maxillary fossa, enters the orbit through the spheno-maxillary fissure, traverses the infra-orbital canal in the floor of the orbit, and appears upon the face at the infra-orbital foramen. At its termination the nerve lies beneath the Levator labii superioris muscle, and divides into a leash of branches, which spread out upon the side of the nose, the lower eyelid, and upper lip, joining with filaments of the facial nerve.

3. The **Inferior Maxillary Nerve** distributes branches to the teeth and gums of the lower jaw, the integument of the temple and external

ear, the lower part of the face and lower lip, and the muscles of mastication; it also supplies the tongue with a large branch. It is the largest of the three divisions of the fifth, and is made up of two roots. Immediately beneath the base of the skull this nerve divides into two trunks, anterior and posterior.

The anterior and small division, which receives nearly the whole of the motor root, divides into branches which supply the muscles of mastication.

The posterior and larger division of the inferior maxillary nerve is for the most part sensory, but receives a few filaments from the motor root. It divides into three branches: the lingual (gustatory) that supplies most of the tongue, the inferior dental, that supplies the teeth and the auriculo-temporal, the only one of these that is concerned with migraine treatment.

The **auricular-temporal** generally arises by two roots, between which the **middle meningeal artery** passes. It runs backward beneath the External pterygoid muscle to the inner side of the neck of the lower jaw. It then turns up with the **temporal artery,** between the external ear and condyle of the jaw, under cover of the parotid gland, and, escaping from beneath this structure, ascends over the zygoma and divides into two temporal branches.

The **Sixth or abducent nerve** supplies the External rectus muscle of the eye. The nerve pierces the dura mater on the basilar surface of the sphenoid bone, runs through a notch immediately below the posterior clinoid process, and enters the cavernous sinus. It passes forward through the sinus, lying on the outer side of the **internal carotid artery.** It enters the orbit through the sphenoidal fissure, and lies above **the ophthalmic vein,** from which it is separated by a lamina of dura mater. It then passes between the two heads of the External rectus, and is distributed to that muscle on its ocular surface.

The **seventh or facial nerve** is the motor nerve of all the muscles of expression in the face, and of the Platysma and Buccinator; the muscles of the External ear; the posterior belly of the Digastric, and the stylo-hyoid. Its chorda tympani branch is the nerve of taste for the anterior two-thirds of the tongue and the vaso-dilator nerve of the submaxillary and sub-lingual glands; its tympanic branch supplies the Stapedius.

The auditory nerve lies to its outer side; and between the two is a small portion of connective tissue which arises from the medulla and joins the facial nerve in the internal auditory meatus.

The facial nerve, firmer and rounder, and smaller than the

auditory, passes forward and outward upon the middle peduncle of the cerebellum, and enters the internal auditory meatus with the auditory nerve. Within the meatus the facial nerve lies in a groove along the upper and anterior part of the auditory nerve, and the pars intermedia is placed between the two, and joins the inner angle of the geniculate ganglion.

At the bottom of the meatus, the facial nerve enters the aquaeductus Fallopii, and follows the course of that canal through the petrous portion of the temporal bone, from its commencement at the internal meatus, to its termination at the stylo-mastoid foramen. It is at first directed outward between the cochlea and vestibule toward the inner wall of the tympanum; it then bends suddenly backwards and arches downwards behind the typanum to the stylo-mastoid foramen.

On emerging from the sterno-mastoid foramen it runs forward in the substance of the parotid gland, **crosses the external carotid artery,** and divides behind the rampus of the lower jaw into two primary branches, temporo-facial and cervico-facial, from which numerous offsets are distributed over the side of the head, face, and upper part of the neck, supplying the superficial muscles in these regions. As the primary branches and their offsets diverge from each other, they present somewhat the appearance of a bird's claw.

It should be noted that at its exit from the stylo-mastoid foramen it communicates with the **pneumogastric nerve.**

Its Branches of Distribution include:—

On the face	Temporo-facial	Temporal Malar Infra-orbital
	Cervico-facial	Buccal Supramaxillary Inframaxillary

The **temporo-facial,** the larger of the two terminal branches, passes upward and forward through the parotid glands, **crosses the external carotid artery and temporo-maxillary vein,** and passes over the neck of the condyle of the jaw, being connected in this situation with the auriculo-temporal branch of the inferior maxillary nerve, and divides into branches which are distributed over the temple and upper part of the face; these are divided into three sets — temporal, malar and infra-orbital.

Of these, the infra-orbital, is larger than the rest, and passes horizontally forwards to be distributed between the lower margin of the orbit and the mouth. The superficial branches run beneath the skin and above the superficial muscles of the face, which they supply: some branches are distributed to the Pyramidalis nasi, joining at the inner angle of the orbit with the infratrochlear and nasal branches of the ophthalmic. The deep branches pass beneath the Zygomatic bone and the upper lip, supplying them and the muscles of the lower orbit, and form a plexus (infraorbital) by joining with the infraorbital branch of the superior maxillary nerve and the buccal branches of the cervico facial.

The **Cervico-facial division of the facial nerve** passes obliquely downward and forward through the parotid gland, **crossing the external carotid artery.** In this situation it is joined by branches from the great auricular nerve. Opposite the angle of the lower jaw it divides into branches which are distributed on the lower half of the face and upper part of the neck.

The **Eighth or Auditory Nerve** is the special nerve of the sense of hearing, being distributed exclusively to the internal ear.

The **Ninth or Glosso-pharyngeal Nerve** is distributed, as its name implies, to the tongue and pharynx, being the nerve of ordinary sensation to the mucous membrane of the pharynx, fauces, and tonsil; and the nerve of taste to all parts of the tongue to which it is distributed.

From its superficial origin it passes outward across the flocculus, and leaves the skull at the central part of the jugular foramen, in a separate sheath of the dura mater, external to and in front of the pneumogastric and spinal accessory nerves. In its passage through the jugular foramen it grooves the lower border of the petrous portion of the temporal bone, and at its exit from the skull passes forward **between the jugular vein and internal carotid artery,** and descends in front of the latter vessel, and beneath the styloid process and the muscles connected with it, to the lower border of the Stylo-pharyngeus. The nerve now crosses inward, forming an arch on the side of the neck, and lying upon the Stylo-pharyngeus and Middle constrictor of the pharynx. It then passes beneath the Hyoglossus, and is finally distributed to the mucous membrane of the fauces and base of the tongue, and the mucous glands of the mouth and tonsil.

The branches of distribution are the tympanic, carotid, pharyngeal, muscular, tonsillar, and lingual.

The **tympanic branch** arises from the petrous ganglion, and enters a small bony canal in the lower surface of the petrous portion of the temporal bone, the lower opening of which is situated on the bony ridge which separates the carotid canal from the jugular fossa. It ascends to the tympanum, enters that cavity by an aperture in its floor close to the inner wall, and divides into branches which are contained in grooves upon the surface of the promontory, forming the tympanic plexus.

The **carotid branches descend along the trunk of the internal carotid artery** as far as its commencement, communicating with the pharyngeal branch of the penumogastric and with branches of the sympathetic.

The **pharyngeal branches** are three of four filaments which unite opposite the middle constrictor of the pharynx with the pharyngeal branches of the pneumogastric and sympathetic nerves to form the pharyngeal plexus, branches from which perforate the muscular coat of the pharynx to supply the muscles and mucous membrane.

The **muscular branch** is distributed to the Stylo-pharyngeus.

The **tonsillar branches** supply the tonsil.

The **lingual branches** are two in number: one supplies the circumvallate papillae and the mucous membrane covering the surface of the base of the tongue; the other perforates its substance, and supplies the mucous membrane and follicular glands of the posterior half of the tongue and communicates with the lingual nerve.

The **tenth or pneumogastric nerve** (vagus nerve) has a more extensive distribution than any of the other cranial nerves passing through the neck and thorax to the upper part of the abdomen. It is composed of both motor and sensory fibres. It supplies the organs of voice and respiration with motor and sensory fibres and the pharynx, **oesophagus and stomach** and heart with motor fibres. Its superficial origin is by eight or ten filaments from the groove between the olivary and the restiform body below the glosso-pharyngeal.

The filaments become united and form a flat cord, which passes outward beneath the flocculus to the jugular foramen, through which it emerges from the cranium. In passing through this opening the penumogastric accompanies the spinal accessory, being contained in the same sheath of dura mater with it, a membranous septum separating them from the glosso-pharyngeal.

The nerve passes vertically down the neck within the sheath of the carotid vessels lying between the **internal carotid artery and internal jugular vein** as far as the thyroid cartilage, **and then between the same vein and the common carotid to the root of the neck.** It is

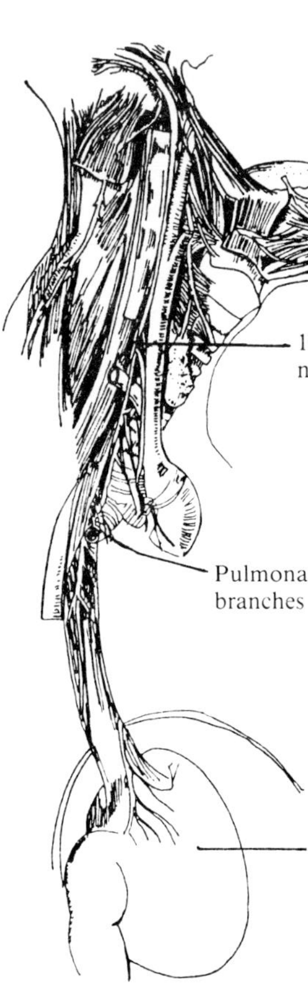

The tenth or pneumogastric nerve.

pressure by the dilated carotid artery on this nerve, supplying the stomach as it does, that contributes to the nausea and vomiting present in the migraine syndrome.

The course of the nerve then becomes different on the two sides of the body. On the right side the nerve passes across the subclavian artery between it and the right innominate vein, and descends by the side of the trachea to the back part of the root of the lung, where it spreads out in a plexiform network from the lower part of which two cords descend upon the oesophagus, on which they divide, forming, with branches from the opposite nerve, the oesophageal plexus (plexus gulae); below, these branches are collected into a single cord, which runs along the back part of the oesophagus, enters the abdomen, and is distributed to the posterior surface of the stomach, joining the left side of the solar plexus, and sending filaments to the splenic plexus and a considerable branch to the coeliac plexus.

On the left side the pneumogastric nerve enters the chest between the left carotid and subclavian arteries, behind the left innominate vein. It crosses the arch of the aorta and descends behind the root of the left lung, forming the posterior pulmonary plexus, and along the anterior surface of the oesophagus, where it unites with the nerve of the right side in forming the oesophageal plexus to the stomach, distributing branches over its anterior surface, some extending over the great cul-de-sac, and others along the lesser curvature. Filaments from these branches enter the gastro-hepatic omentum and join the hepatic plexus.

The branches of the pneumogastric are

In the jugular fossa . . .	Meningeal Auricular
In the neck . . .	Pharyngeal Superior laryngeal Recurrent laryngeal Cervical cardiac
In the thorax . . .	Thoracic cardiac Anterior pulmonary Posterior pulmonary Oesophageal
In the abdomen . . .	Gastric

The meningeal branch is a recurrent filament given off from the ganglion of the root in the jugular foramen. It passes backwards and is distributed to the dura mater covering the posterior fossa of the base of the skull. The auricular branch arises from the ganglion of the root. It divides into two branches, one of which communicates with the posterior auricular nerve, while the other supplies the skin at the back part of the ear and the posterior part of the external auditory meatus.

The pharyngeal branch, the principal motor nerve of the pharynx, arises from the upper part of the inferior ganglion of the pneumogastric.

From the pharyngeal plexus a minute filament is given off, which descends and joins the hypoglossal nerve as it winds round the occipital artery.

The superior laryngeal is the nerve of sensation to the larynx.

The external laryngeal branch gives branches to the pharyngeal plexus and the inferior constrictor, and communicates with the superior cardiac nerve, behind the common carotid.

The internal laryngeal branch supplies the mucous membrane surrounding the superior orifice of the larynx, as well as the membrane which lines the cavity of the larynx as low down as the vocal cord.

The inferior or recurrent laryngeal, so called from its reflected course, is the motor nerve of the larynx.

The recurrent laryngeal, as it winds round the subclavian artery and aorta, gives off several cardiac filaments, which unite with the cardiac branches from the pneumogastric and sympathetic. As it ascends in the neck it gives off oesophageal branches, more numerous on the left than on the right side, which supply the mucous membrane and muscular coat of the oesophagus; tracheal branches to the mucous membrane and muscular fibres of the trachea: and some pharyngeal filaments to the Inferior constrictor of the pharynx.

The cervical cardiac branches, two or three in number, arise from the pneumogastric, at the upper and lower part of the neck.

The superior branches are small, and communicate with the cardiac branches of the sympathetic. They can be traced to the great or deep cardiac plexus. The inferior branches, on one side, arise at the lower part of the neck, just above the first rib. On the right side this branch passes in front or by the side of the arteria innominata, and communicate with one of the cardiac nerves proceeding to the great or deep cardiac plexus. On the left side it passes in front of the arch of the aorta and joins the superficial cardiac plexus.

The thoracic cardiac branches, on the right side, arise from the trunk of the pneumogastric as it lies by the side of the trachea, and from its recurrent laryngeal branch, but on the left side from the recurrent nerve only; passing inward, they terminate in the deep cardiac plexus.

The anterior pulmonary branches, two or three in number, and of small size, are distributed on the anterior aspect of the root of the lungs. They join with filaments from the sympathetic, and form the anterior pulmonary plexus

The posterior pulmonary branches, more numerous and larger than the anterior, are distributed on the posterior aspect of the root of the lung: they are joined by filaments from the third and fourth (sometimes also first and second) thoracic ganglia of the sympathetic, and form the posterior pulmonary plexus. Branches from both plexuses accompany the ramification of the air-tubes through the substance of the lungs.

The **oesophageal branches** are given off from the pneumogastric both above and below the pulmonary branches. The lower are more numerous and larger than the upper. They form, together with branches from the opposite nerve, the oesophageal plexus gulae. From this plexus branches are distributed to the back of the pericardium.

The **gastric branches** are the terminal filaments of the pneumogastric nerve. The nerve on the **right side** is distributed to the **posterior surface** of the stomach, and joins the left side of the coelic plexus and the splenic plexus. The nerve on the **left side** is distributed to the **anterior surface** of the stomach, some filaments passing across the great cul-de-sac, and others along the lesser curvature. They unite with branches of the right nerve and with the sympathetic, some filaments passing through the lesser omentum to the hepatic plexus.

The **eleventh or spinal accessory nerve** consists of two parts, one, the accessory part of the vagus or pneumogastric nerve and the other the spinal portion.

The **bulbar or accessory part** is the smaller of the two. It passes outward to the jugular foramen, where it interchanges fibres with the spinal portion or becomes united to it for a short distance; it is also connected in the foramen, with the upper ganglion of the vagus or pneumogastric nerve by one or two filaments. It then passes through the foramen, and becoming again separated from the spinal portion it is continued over the surface of the ganglion of the trunk of the pneumogastric, being adherent to its surface, and is distributed principally to the pharyngeal and superior laryngeal branches of the pneumogastric. Through the pharyngeal branch it probably supplies the muscles of the soft palate. Some few filaments from it are continued into the trunk of the pneumogastric below the ganglion, to be distributed with the recurrent laryngeal nerve, and probably also with the cardiac nerves.

The **spinal portion** is firm in texture.

This nerve ascends between the ligamentum denticulatum and the posterior roots of the spinal nerves, enters the skull through the foramen magnum, and is **then directed outward to the jugular foramen, through which it passes, lying in the same sheath as the pneumogastric.** In the jugular foramen it receives one or two filaments from the accessory portion. At its exit from the jugular foramen it passes backward, either in front of or behind the **internal jugular vein,** and descends obliquely behind the Digastric and the Stylo-hyoid muscles and pierces the Sterno-mastoid muscle. It passes obliquely across the posterior triangle, to terminate in the deep surface of the Trapezius. This nerve gives several branches to the Sterno-mastoid during its passage through it, and joins in its substance with branches from the second cervical, which supply the muscle. In the posterior triangle it joins with the second and third cervical nerves, while beneath the Trapezius it forms a sort of plexus with the third and fourth cervical nerves, and from this plexus fibres are distributed to the muscle.

The **twelfth or hypoglossal nerve** is the motor nerve of the tongue. The filaments of this nerve are collected into two bundles, which perforate the dura mater separately, opposite the anterior condyloid foramen, and unite together after their passage through it. In those cases in which the anterior condyloid foramen in the occipital bone is double, these two portions of the nerve are separated by a small piece of bone which divides the foramen. The nerve descends almost vertically to a point corresponding with the angle of the jaw. It is at first deeply seated beneath the **internal carotid artery and the internal jugular vein,** and intimately connected with the **pneumogastric nerve.** It then passes forward between the vein and the artery, and lower down in the neck becomes superficial below the Digastric muscle. The nerve then loops round the occipital artery, and crosses the external carotid and its lingual branch below the tendon of the Digastric muscle. It then passes beneath the tendon of the Digastric, the Stylo-hyoid, and the Mylo-hyoid muscles, lying between the last named muscle and the Hyo-glossus, and communicates at the anterior border of the Hyo-glossus with the lingual (gustatory) nerve; it is then continued forward in the fibres of the Genio-hyo-glossus muscle as far as the tip of the tongue, distributing branches to its muscular substance.

The branches of communication are — with the

Pneumogastric	First and second cervical nerves
Sympathetic	Lingual (gustatory)

The branches of distribution are — the

Meningeal	Thyro-hyoid
Descendens hypoglossi	Muscular

Meningeal branches — As the hypoglossal nerve passes through the anterior condyloid foramen it gives off several filaments to the dura mater in the posterior fossa of the base of the skull; these filaments are probably derived from a branch which passes from the first cervical nerve to the hypoglossal nerve.

The **descendens hypoglossi** is a long slender branch, which leaves the hypoglossal where it turns round the **occipital artery.** It consists mainly of fibres which pass to the hypoglossal from the first and second cervical nerves in the above mentioned communication. It descends in front of or within the sheath of the carotid vessels, giving off a branch to the **anterior belly of the omo-hyoid,** and then joins the communicating branches from the second and third cervical nerves, just below the middle of the neck, to form a loop, the ansa hypoglossi. From the convexity of this loop branches pass to supply the Sterno-hyoid, Sterno-thyroid, and the **posterior belly of the omo-hyoid.** Another filament descends in front of the vessels into the chest, and joins the cardiac and phrenic nerves.

The **thyro-hyoid** is a small branch arising from the hypoglossal near the posterior border of the Hyo-glossus; it passes obliquely across the great cornu of the hyoid bone and supplies the Thyro-hyoid muscle.

The muscular branches are distributed to the Stylo-glossus, Hyoglossus, Genio-hyoid, and Genio-hyo-glossus muscles. At the under surface of the tongue numerous slender branches pass upward into the substance of the organ to supply its intrinsic muscles.

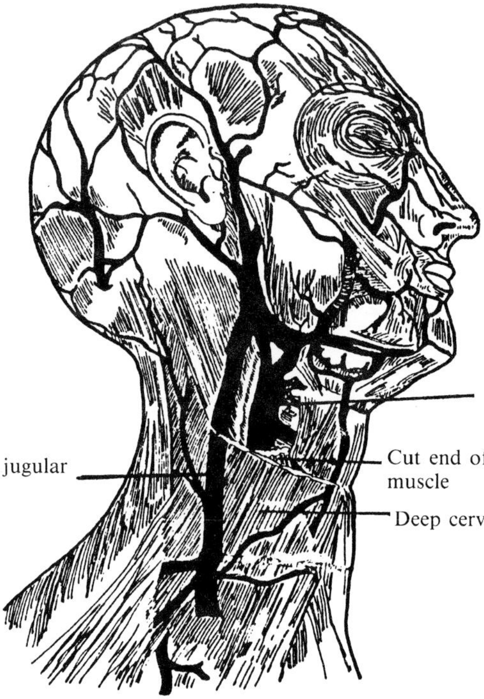

The veins of the head and neck.

The Veins of the Head and Neck

VEINS are the vessels which serve to return the blood from the capillaries of the different parts of the body to the heart. Veins are larger and more numerous than arteries. In form they are perfectly cylindrical but slight constructions occur at intervals indicating the existence of valves in their interior. To enable free communication between veins often large and frequent anastomoses occur especially in the cavity of the cranium and between the veins of the neck where any obstruction would be dangerous to the cerebral venous system. Veins have thinner walls than arteries with less elasticity.

Generally speaking, only the veins of the head and neck are of real importance in the treatment of migraine. All superficial veins of the face, neck and side of the head enter the **external jugular** vein, whereby the venous blood is carried to the heart and then to the lungs for re-oxygenation of the blood cells. Similarly the venous returns from the brain are carried by the **internal jugular** vein to the heart and pumped by the heart to the lungs for re-oxygenation.

If the head is held in forward flexion for considerable periods of time the **external** jugular vein may be caught up in a fold of skin and the superficial fascia of the neck causing some interference of the venous blood flow via the vein. This causes some dilatation of most of the veins of the face and head, particularly the temporal veins which may stand out prominently.

If the posture of the head and neck is sufficient to cause moderate pressure on the **internal** jugular vein then slight cerebral congestion will result, leading to a light-headed sensation with some dizziness. It must be noted that this can occur without necessarily pressure being exerted on the common carotid artery to cause a complete migraine syndrome. However pressure on the internal jugular vein usually causes the first symptoms of a migraine attack. Greater prolonged forward flexion of the head causes pressure by the tendon of the omohyoid muscle on the cervical fascia which encloses the internal jugular vein, the common carotid artery and the pneumogastric nerve. This leads to the full migraine syndrome.

The veins of the head and neck may be subdivided into three groups:

1. The veins of the exterior of the head and face.
2. The veins of the neck.
3. The veins of the diploe and the interior of the cranium.

Only the first two groups will be described in detail, as they only are relevant to the discussion on migraine treatment.

1. Veins of the Exterior of the Head and Face

The veins of the exterior of the head and face are:

Frontal	Temporal
Supra-orbital	Occipital
Angular	Internal Maxillary
Facial	Temporo-maxillary
	Posterior auricular

Of these, five only will be described in more detail

a) The frontal vein
b) The supra-orbital vein
c) The facial vein
d) The temporal vein
e) The occipital vein

a) **The Frontal Vein** commences on the anterior part of the skull by a venous plexus which communicates with the anterior tributaries of the temporal vein. The veins converge to form a single trunk, which runs downwards near the middle line of the forehead parallel with the vein of the opposite side, and unites with it at the root of the nose, by a transverse branch, called the nasal arch. Occasionally the frontal veins join to form a single trunk, which bifurcates at the root of the nose into the two angular veins. At the root of the nose the veins diverge, and join the supra-orbital vein, at the inner angle of the orbit, to form the angular vein.

b) **The Supra-orbital Vein** commences on the forehead, communicating with the anterior temporal vein, and runs downwards and inwards, superficial to the occipito-frontalis muscle, receiving tributaries from the neighbouring structures, and joins the frontal vein at the inner angle of the orbit to form the angular vein.

c) **Facial Vein.** The facial vein commences at the side of the root of the nose, being a direct continuation of the angular vein. It lies behind and follows a less tortuous course than the facial artery. It passes obliquely downwards and outwards, and crosses over the body of the lower jaw, with the facial artery, and, passing obliquely outwards and backwards, beneath the Platysma and cervical fascia, unites with the anterior division of the temporo-maxillary vein to form a trunk of large size (common facial vein) which enters the internal jugular. From near its termination a communicating branch often runs down the anterior border of the Sterno-mastoid to join the lower part of the anterior jugular.

d) **Temporal Vein.** The temporal vein commences by a minute plexus on the side and vertex of the skull, which communicates with the frontal and supra-orbital veins in front, the corresponding vein of the opposite side, and the posterior auricular and occipital veins behind. From this network, anterior and posterior branches are formed which unite to form the trunk of the vein. This trunk is joined in this situation by a large vein, the middle temporal, which receives the blood from the substance of the Temporal muscle and pierces the fascia at the upper border of the zygoma. The temporal vein then descends between the external auditory meatus and the condoyle of the jaw, enters the substance of the parotid gland, and unites with the internal maxillary vein to form the temporo-maxillary vein.

Tributaries — The temporal vein receives in its course some parotid veins, an articular branch from the articulation of the jaw, anterior auricular veins from the external ear, and a vein of large size, the transverse facial, from the side of the face. The middle temporal vein, previous to its junction with the temporal vein, receives a branch, the orbital vein, which is formed by some external palpebral branches, and passes backwards between the layers of the temporal fascia.

e) **The Occipital Veins** commence at the back of the vertex of the skull, by a plexus, in a similar manner to the other veins. **These unite to form one or two veins, which follow the course of the occipital artery, passing deeply between the muscle of the back part of the neck, and terminate in the internal jugular,** occasionally in the external jugular vein. As these veins pass across the mastoid portion of the temporal bone, one of them receives the mastoid vein, and thus establishes a communication with the lateral sinus.

2. Veins of the Neck

The veins of the neck, which return the blood from the head and face, are the

External jugular	Anterior jugular
Posterior external jugular	Internal jugular

and Vertebral, though the latter is not relevant here.

a) **The External Jugular Vein** receives the greater part of the blood from the exterior of the cranium and deep parts of the face, being formed by the junction of the posterior division of the temporo-maxillary with the posterior auricular vein. It commences in the substance of the parotid gland, on a level with the angle of the lower jaw, and runs perpendicularly down the neck, in the direction of a line drawn from the angle of the jaw to the middle of the clavicle. In its courses it crosses the Sterno-mastoid muscle, and runs parallel with its posterior border as far as its attachment to the clavicle, where it perforates the deep fascia, and terminates in the subclavian vein, on the outer side of, or in front of, the Scalenus anticus muscle. In the neck it is separated from the sterno-mastoid by the investing layer of the deep cervical fascia, and is covered by the Platysma, the superficial fascia, and the integument or skin.

The external jugular vein varies in size, bearing an inverse proportion to that of the other veins of the neck; it is occasionally double. It is provided with two pairs of valves, the lower pair being placed at the entrance into the subclavian vein, the upper pair in most cases about an inch and a half above the clavicle. The portion of vein between the two sets of valves is often dilated, and is termed the sinus. These valves do not prevent the regurgitation of the blood, or the passage of injection from below upwards.

b) **The Posterior External Jugular Vein.** The posterior external jugular vein commences in the occipital region and returns the blood from the integument and superficial muscles in the upper and back part of the neck, lying between the Splenius and Trapezius muscles. It runs down the back part of the neck, and opens into the external jugular just below the middle of its course.

c) **The Anterior Jugular Vein.** The anterior jugular vein commences near the hyoid bone from the convergence of several superficial veins from the submaxillary region. It passes down between the median line and the anterior border of the Sterno-mastoid, and, at the lower part of the neck, passes beneath that muscle to open into the termination of the external jugular, or into the subclavian vein. This vein varies considerably in size, bearing almost always an inverse proportion to the external jugular. Most frequently there are two anterior jugulars, right and left; but occasionally only one. This vein received some laryngeal veins, and occasionally a small thyroid vein. Just above the sternum, the two anterior jugular veins communicate by a transverse trunk, which receives tributaries from the inferior thyroid veins. It also communicates with the internal jugular. There are no valves in this vein.

d) **The Internal Jugular Vein.** The internal jugular vein collects the blood from the interior of the cranium, from the superficial parts of the face, and from the neck. It commences just external to the jugular foramen, at the base of the skull, being formed by the coalescence of the lateral and inferior petrosal sinuses. At its origin it is somewhat dilated, and this dilatation is called the sinus, or bulb, of the internal jugular vein. It runs down the side of the neck in a vertical direction, **lying at first on the outer side of the internal carotid, and then on the outer side of the common carotid,** and at the root of the neck unites with the subclavian vein to form the innominate vein. The internal jugular vein, at its commencement, lies upon the Rectus capitis lateralis, **and behind the internal carotid artery and the nerves passing through the jugular foramen; lower down the vein and artery lie upon the same plane, the glosso-pharyngeal and hypoglossal nerves passing forwards between them; the pneumogastric descends between and behind them in the same sheath,** and the spinal accessory passes obliquely outwards, behind or in front of the vein. At the root of the neck the vein of the right side is placed at a little distance from the artery, on the left side it usually lies over the artery at its lower part. The right internal jugular vein crosses the first part of the subclavian artery. The vein is of considerable size, but varies in different individuals, the left one being usually the smaller. It is provided with a pair of valves, which are placcd at its point of termination, or from half to three-quarters of an inch above it.

APPENDIX B

I HAVE included here several recent case histories of my patients. In most cases they have been written by the patients themselves and copied with very little editing — if at all. Whilst they show that my treatment is effective, they are reproduced primarily to give readers some idea of the nature of the migraine syndrome from a sufferer's point of view, the effect it has on people's lives and the frustration of the patient who has repeatedly sought help that is not currently available in present day medicine.

Case History I

Heather McFarlane
18 McBeth
Calderwood
East Kilbride

This patient is a young girl, 13 years old. Her parents were present at each treatment in my surgery and were more than willing to write up Heather's history for me. The story speaks for itself.

October, 1988

Doctor (1)

SYMPTOMS — Headache, sore throat, sickness. Diagnosed as viral infection. TREATMENT — Penicillin V and Paracetamol. Ten days after this treatment Heather was taken to see a doctor who prescribed continuing Paracetamol as cause of problem was due to her age.

Doctor (2)

One week later Heather paid further visit to doctor who was informed of blurred vision and flashes in the eyes, as well as severe headache and sickness. During this period Heather's appetite had faded totally. This was an extremely worrying point as her appetite had always been healthy. On this visit doctor recommended Heather have an eye test. Next day optician tested her eyes and prescribed glasses as her eyes had deteriorated considerably since August and this was now November (2).

On obtaining glasses Heather returned to school but was sent home after being sick and complaining of headache. Further visit to doctor was made, who said in his opinion eight Paracetamol per day was quite all right as problem was a recurring viral infection. When informed that Paracetamol was doing no good, doctor prescribed Sofradex ear drops.

At this point Heather's mother asked to be referred to a specialist. Reluctantly this was agreed. Unfortunately, she is still waiting as appointment is for May, 1989.

Doctor (3)

Heather returns to school. Up to this point she had been spending most of her time in bed in darkened room.

Once more she is sent home from school.

Further visit to doctor was made who, on being informed of past treatment, suggested this was an allergy and prescribed Beconase nasal spray and Polysporn ear drops and to continue with Paracetamol. An appointment for following week was made and on this visit doctor suggested it might be migraine, and prescribed Paramax, four per day. No TV or VDU screens, no swimming or discos with flashing lights and a further appointment one week later. On this visit told to continue with Beconase and Paramax, also given Galpsend Linctus and told to phone for repeat prescriptions as required, and doctor would see her in four weeks.

This is now January, 1989

After a chance conversation with friend who mentioned the migraine treatment she and her mother had received from A. Walker-Naddell we decided to contact him. On first visit Heather described symptoms. Mr. Naddell's opinion was that it was migraine. After receiving her first treatment Heather was able for the first time in three months to abstain from all painkilling drugs and sprays.

On each progressive visit Heather's appetite and general well being has improved dramatically to say the least. To date Heather has not taken any painkilling drug.

During this treatment both myself and my wife have been present and to say Mr. Walker-Naddell's treatment is successful would be the understatement of the decade.

James & Elspeth McFarlane (signed)

Case History 2

Marie Corish

737 Mosspark Drive
Cardonald
Glasgow

This account was written by the patient herself and tells the story of a young lifetime of suffering and missed opportunities.

Age 10	*Fainted in playground playing skipping ropes.*
10-11	*Fainted every four months, feeling dizzy, weakness in legs.*
11	*Migraine headaches and fainting — G.P. said not to worry because I would grow out of it (puberty) and probably not hurt myself.*
11	*Attend Yorkhill Children's Hospital — Head Professor prescribed Phenobarbatel for pain, said I would grow out of fainting but I would have migraine headaches for the next 40 years. I had my first E.E.G. because they thought I might have epilepsy — however they could not find conclusive evidence of epilepsy although they did not discount it altogether.*
13-16	*Attended Southern General Hospital under Dr. Draper's clinic. Tested with E.E.G. and E.C.G. because they thought it may be connected with my heart.* *Fainting frequently, missed a lot of school.* *Again doctors said it was my age and I would grow out of it.* *Doctors said I was bringing it upon myself whenever I couldn't handle a situation.*

My father died when I was seven and we emigrated from Canada to Scotland when I was eight leaving my older brother behind. They said this had an emotional effect on me and was deep in my subconscious.

18 *Had an operation for a cyst on my left ovary. G.P. said that the build-up of this may have been the cause of my fainting, nausea and dizziness. They hoped that after this operation the fainting would stop — it did not.*

Throughout school and different jobs, every time I studied for exams I tended to faint more, so much so that I was advised that it would be better if I didn't go to University.

19 *Moved to Manchester. Company I worked for were concerned and recommended further investigation as I hurt myself on a computer when I fell during a faint. They diagnosed that I was getting worked up about things and when this happened my blood pressure would drop causing me to faint. During normal times my blood pressure was low but not sufficient to warrant medication.*

I returned to Glasgow — did not seek employment as I was fainting very regularly. G.P. recommended I go back to the Southern General and see a psychiatrist. G.P. still felt fainting was due to death of father at an early age. Had three sessions with psychiatrist — told me there was nothing wrong with me and I did not need his help.

20 *Had to give up new job as company were concerned about my safety at work (lots of stairs). Doctors said the only thing they could do was put me in hospital for tests until they found something. I was fitted with a heart monitor (mobile E.C.G.) Did not faint while it was fitted. They discovered that when I felt dizzy and faint one pupil was dilated more than the other but could not give any reason for it or suggest how this might cause fainting.*

21 *Now working in Edinburgh for a year. Off work every month with fainting or depression. I slept a lot and stayed in a lot. I was taking a lot of time off work but the doctors kept telling me there was nothing wrong with me and I was bringing it upon myself. My Manager was angry that I was taking a lot of time off work and therefore there was more pressure on me causing me to get even more depressed and faint. I was also told that I had an ulcer and to eat Rennies, Settlers etc. whenever I had a sore stomach.*

22 *Taken off the Pill — said it was the cause of my migraines.*

Told to have a baby — this would solve all the problems.

Told my wisdom teeth were cause of migraine as they were giving me a lot of pain and trouble.

22-23 *Returned to Glasgow, felt more relaxed at home and I was now very settled (recently married). However the fainting, weakness, dizziness and nausea returned. I went to a hypnotherapist to see if he could make me relax. At this stage I was beginning to believe that I was in fact bringing it all upon myself and that something in my past was making me strained and anxious. The hypnotherapist said that he would be able to make me relax to get to the root of the problem, which he also felt was the death of my father. I attended his clinic for a month and although I was more relaxed and confident in the short term, I was still fainting.*

A friend of my mother had been seen by Mr. Walker-Naddell about her spinal problems and sore legs. After a few appointments she was feeling as though she had a new back and new legs. She strongly recommended Mr. Walker-Naddell.

At my first session Mr. Walker-Naddell said the cause of my sore heads, fainting etc. was caused by muscles in my neck. I have felt a big difference since attending his clinic, as if a cloud had been lifted off my shoulders. I was told to disregard previous treatments — not to take Mygril or Distilgesic or Panstan Forte (for pain). I've no longer to lie in a dark room.

Since starting his treatment I have felt considerably better, more energetic and have not been fainting. Mr. Walker-Naddell is confident that I will be cured completely but at this stage I may still suffer some dizziness etc. until the treatment is finished. This in fact has been the case.

SYMPTOMS OF A FAINT

— *Generally no warning*
— *Occasionally felt dizzy and sick beforehand (sore stomach)*
— *Faint*
— *Usually out for at least 15-30 minutes*
— *When out completely unaware of surroundings*
— *Cannot be brought out of a faint — have to come out on my own*

— *Afterwards very upset, sore head, cold hands and feet, tingling in hands*
— *Very tired and weak afterwards, need to sleep*

Later Letter

I have been visiting Mr. Walker-Naddell for the past two months and I feel like a different person. I have been able to live a more normal life and can arrange engagements without the worry of not being able to fulfil them.

I feel that a weight has been lifted off my shoulders and can cope with pressures of work without fainting or having to leave work with a migraine headache. I have more energy for my daily life without a dark cloud hanging over my head.

Since the age of 11 going into a dark room and taking painkillers has been my only cure for one of my attacks, now I am convinced that if I continue with my exercises I have nothing to worry about and my attack, if any, will disappear.

I am very grateful to Mr. Walker-Naddell because I think my future in my present job wouldn't be as secure nor would my outlook have changed so much.

Thanks to Mr. Walker-Naddell I feel that I can tackle anything.

Case History 3

Mrs. M. Fitzsimmons

5 Melvick Place
Glasgow G51 4P

This story of migraine starts when the patient is a mature woman but nevertheless she has endured constantly recurring pain for 17 years. The migraine-type headache in this case has been caused as a direct result of a cervical disc lesion, which, in turn, caused muscle spasm and atrophy and thereby faulty cervical posture.

I have suffered from severe headaches and pain at back of my neck for the past 17 years, the pain at times made me feel ill and I was reduced to tears on most occasions.

When the pain in neck and headaches first started I was about 39 years old. They got so bad I went to my G.P. and was told it was just wear and tear of the discs in my neck and eyestrain that was causing the headaches. They were so severe it was unbearable, so much so I requested a second opinion as all my G.P. could give me were painkilling tablets, which after a while upset my stomach.

I waited some time before I received an appointment to see the Orthopeadic Consultant at the Southern General Hospital.

On the day of the appointment he listened to what I had to say, and then sent me along for x-rays, result! I was referred to the Physiotherapy Dept. where I was put on traction, heat treatment and exercise course three days a week for four weeks. After all that, the pain remained. The hospital's only reply was, all we can offer now is that you wear a surgical collar which they supplied at the end of their treatment. This left me feeling worse than when I first started. The pain continued and in January, 1989 I was forced to go back to my G.P. who once again sent me for x-rays, which resulted in me being told I had arthritis in my neck, and once again told to take Paracetamol for pain.

By chance I was discussing my problem with a friend at work who advised I should visit Mr. A. Walker-Naddell, as he had helped him in the past. He was a football player at that time. I phoned Mr. Naddell's surgery that day and was given an appointment for 3rd March, 1989. (A date I will remember for the rest of my life.) You see after that appointment I felt I had been given a new lease of life.

I am unable to express my gratitude to this gentleman. On my arrival at his surgery in Sandyford Place, Mr. Naddell greeted me and took me into the surgery where I explained what had been wrong with me. First he told me not to wear the collar the hospital had given me. He then proceeded to examine my neck and my head. After a few minutes he told me exactly what was wrong: a disc had moved and was pressing on a nerve. I was given a local anaesthetic and he gently broke off the protruding disc and he then gently treated my head.

How can you express how it feels after all the years of suffering that pain, and after 10 minutes with Mr. Naddell the pain stopped immediately. He did in 10 minutes what a Hospital failed to do in 17 years.

Once again Mr. Naddell, my sincere thanks to you, and may God keep you safe and well to continue your work for people who have been suffering like me.

Yours sincerely

Margaret Fitzsimmons (signed)

P.S. Please let me know when your new book is published.

Case History 4

Una Orlandi

44 Parnell Street
Limerick
Ireland

This case history, again written by the patient herself, gives a vivid and personal description of the symptoms of migraine and the unsuccessful series of tests and treatments that failed to cure it.

Una Orlandi — Age 32 years

Having had treatment from Mr. Naddell I now realise that I have been a sufferer of 'Migraine' for years without knowing the cause of the headaches and dizziness.

Going back to my schooldays I used to faint quite frequently. On seeing our local doctor to see what was causing the headaches he advised my mum to have my hair cut (which was to my waistline) as he felt all of my strength was being lost in the growth of the hair. Carrying out his advice greatly upset me and my mum, as the long natural curls of my hair was her pride and joy. Alas the headaches continued. I was 14 years old.

I became engaged to be married in February, 1983. During the months leading up to my wedding day I continued experiencing severe headaches and a heaviness in my head. I recall one evening the headache being so bad I couldn't move my head from side to side. When I tried to lie down on one side the other side of my head felt as if it was tumbling down. The pain was so bad I felt as if I were going to throw up. I couldn't think or see properly. At midnight I was taken to hospital where a series of lumbar punctures were carried out. The results were normal. After four days I was sent home, told to take some tablets and lie in a dark room. The headaches continued.

I married in August of that year and my husband and I opened our own restaurant. We both worked hard doing long hours and the headaches got worse and worse. Within a year I started having occasional blackouts and returned to my G.P. This time painkillers were prescribed. Within a few weeks I had an open prescription for the tablets but the headaches got worse and worse and I started experiencing severe pain over my right eye and a burning sensation at the back of my neck and between my shoulder blades. The discomfort was unbearable. I became agitated, bad humoured and frustrated as I couldn't carry out the day's work I was used to doing.

At this point I was eight months pregnant. I got up one morning and as I put my feet on the ground I collapsed. I had no feeling in my right side. I was taken to hospital and kept for observation. They advised me that the baby was lying on the nerve, causing the numbness in my arm and leg. I was confined to bed in the hospital for the next two weeks and at this point they induced me and my son was born some hours later. I remember waking up and trying to move my arm and fingers. The pins and needles and tingling in the fingers were still present. Within a week I was advised to see a Neurologist in Cork. I gave him the history of the headaches and pins and needles and next day I was admitted to Cork Regional Hospital. I underwent a series of severe tests for the next six days, lumbar punctures, milogram, nerve condition tests, cat scan, E.E.G.'s. All the results were normal. The final diagnosis was "cervical neuritis". I was sent home, given a prescription for more painkillers which were so strong I couldn't take them as they made me throw up. For the past two years I have had constant headaches, burning between my shoulder blades and severe lower backache which prevents me from sitting down. The pain and cloudiness has become so much a part of me that I cannot remember when I didn't have it. And then I heard about Mr. Walker-Naddell in Scotland.

My husband who has also suffered with me for the past two years decided it was our last chance, so here we are. Tomorrow is my last day of treatment. (Una came on the 3-day 'crash course' available for patients who live at a distance — Ed.) *I haven't had a headache since Tuesday. I still have a lot of discomfort in my lower back and my complete system feels exhausted but I feel that I have reached the end of the road.*

We are ever grateful,

Luigi and Una Orlandi

Case History 5

Kathleen Taylor

The Rowans
11 Drumbeg Loan
Killearn
Glasgow G63 9LG

This case history describes how the onset of migraine symptoms began as a result of a fall and reinforces my theory that migraine is the result of faulty posture or cervical disorders.

With reference to our telephone conversation this morning, I have pleasure in enclosing a brief note of my recovery to date, as you requested.

I will telephone you within the next few weeks to arrange a final consultation. In the meantime, I would like to take this opportunity of thanking you most sincerely for all your kindness and careful attention during the last three months. Before consulting you, I felt I was doomed to a life of constant headaches and neck pains. However, ever since my first visit to you, you have transformed my afflictions as surely as night follows day. I know I join a privileged list of patients who will always be eternally grateful to you.

Yours sincerely,

Kathleen Taylor

Age — 50 years

Problem — Fall, followed by vomiting, leading to the following symptoms.

Symptoms	*Sore head, neck, whiplash, balance unsteady, vision, memory, concentration affected, etc.*
Case History	*I had a virus infection which started on 20th May, 1988 and has been identified as 'coxsackie 'B' virus' following a blood test.* *A week later, I collapsed in my kitchen and fell on my left side. When I came round I found myself vomiting uncontrollably. After being given an injection by my doctor the vomiting ceased. My fall has left me with an extremely sore head especially behind my left ear, where I must have hit the floor — also across the base of the skull and top of my neck. My left ear feels peculiar, slightly blocked, with a numb sensation and crackles on swallowing and moving my jaw. I also have dry eyes from time to time and pain in my forehead over my eyes and very occasionally slight nausea. My balance, vision, concentration, memory etc. have all been affected by my fall. My hands tingle and seem clumsy sometimes, when doing any housework, writing etc. and my co-ordination is also affected.*

Conditions prevailed for one year.

Visted Mr. Naddell in April, 1989 who diagnosed a cervical disc lesion, whiplash, cervical spondylosis and migraine syndrome.

Treatment over a three month period, including non-surgical detachment of the disc under local anaesthesia. After three consultations and daily exercise routine, I began to feel some improvement in all symptoms of disturbed balance, nausea, distorted vision and severe headaches at base of skull leading up over forehead. Within six weeks I felt a definite improvement in all areas, especially the severe headaches which were vastly improved. By the end of a three month period I can say, without doubt, that all the symptoms have almost disappeared. I continue to do my exercise routine twice daily and my headaches, which were constant, are now only occasional.

Case History 6

Mr. J. G. Dawes

55 Legbourne Road
Louth
Lincolnshire
LN11 8ES

This is the story of a man who having endured innumerable unsuccessful courses of treatment was eventually told his condition was psychosomatic and referred to a psychiatrist and indeed spent some months in a mental hospital. What an indictment of contemporary medicine that a man suffering from a physical disorder should be sent to a mental hospital!

Here as you requested is an evaluation of my problems and treatment up until the time I came to see you in March, 1989. The dates are a loose approximation, the onset of symptoms are to the best of my knowledge in the correct order.

Symptom	***Diagnosis/Treatment***
SUMMER 1980 — Onset of pain in left chest, slight nausea, tingling in lips.	*E.C.G. Pulse and blood tests. No results.*

WINTER 1980 — Continuation of chest pain. Some spinal pain, onset of ache under lower right rib. Visual problems and continuing slight nausea.	*Aludrox given for nausea.*
1981 — Symptoms continue.	*Hospital consultant diagnoses Fibrositis as cause of chest pain.*
1982 — Symptoms continue.	*Aludrox given for nausea. Gall bladder x-ray negative. Duodenal ulcer x-ray positive. Ulcer treated, tests show fully healed, pain continues.*
WINTER 1982 — Onset of neck/head pain.	
FEBRUARY 1983 — Some restriction of head movement, head and neck very painful. Hearing affected, nausea, visual problems, tingling arms and hands. Felt dreadful.	*Painkillers. PSYCHIATRIC TREATMENT.*
JULY 1983 — All problems continue, although chest a little better. Head bad, and seems bloated.	*Discharged from RAF. NOT ON MEDICAL GROUNDS. End of normal engagement. Discharged as being in good health.*

Now with a civilian practitioner after RAF service.

SUMMER 1983 — Head/neck pain continue. Nausea, visual problems. Some hearing troubles. Feel dreadful.	*Painkillers. Medicine for nausea.*
WINTER 1983 — As above.	*Hospital consultant (Louth) diagnoses depression. More pills.*

Symptoms	*Diagnosis/Treatment*
1984 — Symptoms continue although chest less troublesome.	*Throughout the year painkillers, Beta-blockers, stomach medicine.*
1985 — Symptoms continue.	*Hospital consultant (Hull). Brain scan. No result. Diagnosed as being psychosomatic.*
1985/86 — REFERRED TO PSYCHIATRIST. With same continuing.	*DIAGNOSED EPILEPSY. Mental hospital two months.*
SUMMER 1986 — Head pain, visual problems, some neck pain, tingling hands and arms. Some nausea pain/ discomfort below lower right rib. Referred to London.	*National Hospital for Nervous Diseases. Consultant diagnosed chronic muscular tension. Treated with pills, over 18 month period. Included 10 day stay in hospital. Many x-rays, blood tests. Nothing found.*
LATE 1987 — Symptoms continue as above.	*Course of treatment with an Osteopath. No results.*
	Course of treatment with Acupuncture. No results.
JANUARY 1988 — Symptoms continue as above but head very bad.	*Visited a physiotherapist. Informed spine bent to right 7/12th vertebrae.*
1988 — Symptoms continue but head very, very bad.	*Had approximately 40 treatments on weekly basis. Spine straightened, pain eased. Unable to convince G.P. that spine may be cause of trouble.*

Success at third request, referred to Orthopaedic surgeon Louth Hospital.

SEPTEMBER, 1988 — *Blood tests, x-ray of spine (lying down). No results. Surgeon diagnosed depression.*

1989 — Through Mrs. Adams (Physio) I heard of you, and it was in hope and desperation that I wrote to you in March.

I hope this information is of some help to you. Some of the details are becoming a little hazy but the core of problem is here.

Yours sincerely

J. G. Dawes (45 years)

I am still carrying out the exercises thoroughly four/five times a day, and I would say that I feel better for doing so. Considering that I have suffered with this for eight years or so three weeks is probably not sufficient time to right all the wrongs. I do, however, feel confident that this approach will eventually win through.

I will write to you again in about three weeks and give you a further update on progress.

Yours sincerely,

J. G. Dawes (signed)

(No news is good news! Ed.)

Case History 7

A. M. Walker
14 Dalziel Drive,
Pollokshields
Glasgow G41 4PT

October, 1989

When I read Jack Webster's item in the Herald in April, in which he described your theory of postural migraine syndrome, I was, I confess, hopeful if a little sceptical.

I first experienced migraine at the age of 32 shortly after I started taking the "pill". At the time, the journals were carrying many reports of oral-contraceptive-related conditions, including headache. I stopped taking the pill, the headaches continued . . . I am now 52 years old and have had prescribed just about every specific migraine treatment from the ergots to beta-blockers. The painkillers and vaso-contructors gave symptomatic relief and prophylactics worked for limited periods of time. Latterly, nothing had any appreciable effect and therefore I took nothing! In these 20 years, I don't think I experienced more than four consecutive weeks that were migraine-free, and for at least the last ten years, I know there was a causal factor in the neck pain I experienced. I failed, however, to convince my family Doctor of the connection; they were very attentive, but insisted on treating the separate conditions.

It won't be difficult for you to understand the mixed feelings of excitement, optimism and desperation with which people like me greet reports of a "new cure". It is, therefore, with the very greatest sincerity that I can report a quite remarkable improvement since I just consulted you.

On my first visit you confirmed that the migraine syndrome was caused by a prolapsed disc in my cervical spine and, under local anaesthetic, you detached the disc non-surgically. The effect was magical — I realise now that there must have been a degree of constant pain present because when the anaesthetic wore off the "painlessness" was tangible!

I have been carrying out the training programme conscientiously since then and, although I have had about three severe migraine attacks, I have been able to relate these to postural problems, for example, painting a ceiling!

The quality of my life has improved immeasurably — and without drugs. For that, thank you.

Yours sincerely,

A. M. WALKER (Signed)
(Assistant Chief Area Nursing Officer with the Lanarkshire Health Board.)